SECRETS OF AN OVER 50 FORMER FAT MAN

SCOTT DEUTY

DEDICATION

This book is dedicated to Heavenly for her support and the happiness she has added to my life.

I'd like to extend the dedication to my two sons, Michael and Tyler. I haven't always been there physically due to the selfishness of others and due to circumstances beyond my control. I have always been there mentally. I love you boys (now men).

CONTENTS

List of Figures

List of Tables

ACKNOWLEDGMENTS

There is no doubt in my mind that the success I have achieved in life is due to the teachings established by Vince Lombardi. As a young boy, I read everything I could about him and how he brought the Green Bay Packers from a cellar dweller to a team that dominated nearly a decade in the NFL. His teachings instilled within me the drive I needed to start at guard even though I was the second lightest guy on the varsity football team. I also employed the same drive in obtaining my Master's degree as well as pursuing the weight loss that was instrumental in writing this book.

The teachings of Vince Lombardi would not have had the effect they did if it were not for them being implemented by Bart Starr to establish a successful career and shared with audiences through the writing of Jerry Kramer. I thank both of you.

Note that sports figures are not my heroes. Some are inspirations. Anyone who has served in the United States military is my hero. I thank you graciously for giving me the right to freedom of speech as well as protecting that right. Without it, this book would not have been possible.

I also wish to thank my Facebook family who has tolerated my nine months of posting my weight loss progress. I know it wasn't always easy reading however I kept my sanity by having a venue where I could share my success.

FORWARD

The whole purpose for writing a book is so that people will read it. I asked myself why people would want to read this book. The answer was simple. They want an easy and fun way to lose weight and tone up. They also want to know they can succeed in achieving their goal. If the journey is too difficult or painful, no one will want to try it. I must provide a solution to their desires that is achievable, easy, and enjoyable.

Those seem like marketable attributes that will interest readers. But what do people really want in life? Happiness. I was granted the unexpected yet greatly appreciated gift of happiness as a result of my weight loss journey. Walk beside me and find out how.

In the sea of material on weight loss and fitness, no one has documented the success I had in producing the body they always wanted especially when you consider I'm over 50. My journey was so fun and so much easier than I ever imagined. My body was capable of responding in ways I never thought possible. I want to alert you to your own capabilities and share my success with you in a format that is easy to read. I tell you how to lose weight and tone up in a narrated story format that follows my successful journey as it unfolded. By doing so, I wanted to capture your attention in an interesting descriptive narration that could be coming from you the reader as much as from me the author. I write as though you are the main character. Other fitness books use a different approach by instructing you and thus talking down to you. My writing style enables you to walk in my shoes and succeed while being entertained along the way.

This journey benefited me in ways that I never imagined. What started out as an effort to make me physically appealing to others resulted in success and happiness beyond anything I envisioned. I became a much better person overall, not just physically.

I can tell you that a toned body will make people much more aware of you and draw them to you. There was however an amazing transformation in my personality that was the real reason people were drawn to me. I became much happier. It is unbelievable how happiness lowers walls so that people can enter your life. I have gained so many new friends and a close female partner who was extremely happy when I met her. We became close because I enhanced her happiness and she enhances mine.

Imagine that, making a very happy person happier. Who'd "thunk" that fitness and an improved physique would enable that? It did. I'm living proof. I live the dream every day with this exciting woman who is the pinnacle of happiness. I dig watching people flock to her due to an ever present smile.

This book does have a dark side that has a happy ending. I almost canned the whole project when I saw this. I salvaged the effort because there was a very valuable lesson in my learnings. Not only am I providing a happy way to a better body, I'm revealing what success has done to improve me as a person. People and even products are successful because they provide something the public in general desires. Actors perform roles that make us feel good, musicians provide catchy tunes that please us, artists produce visually appealing creations, and athletes perform physical acts of amazement that we envy.

Whereas happiness draws people to us, acting vain repels them. Like it or not, I initially was vain about my accomplishments. This is very apparent throughout the book and especially in the part about motivation. I don't like that person I was nor do I expect you to like him. I have matured beyond that person.

When I started this journey I was motivated to create an exceptional body. This drove me to look better and better as the fat melted away and the physique emerged. What I learned about the human spirit is that physical is only a bridge to the mental. Sure the physique turned heads however if there was a scowl on my face, then who would make the effort to talk to me? The key lesson is that the smile that appeared is what really opened up opportunities. Being fit enabled a happy personality that others found attractive.

Physical appeal is just a natural selection calling card that all species use as method for improving the next generation. We are drawn to the perfect body. This is very apparent in Hollywood actors, and with models and body builders. Herein lies the problem and the lesson I learned. A good body doesn't make a desirable human. One must supplement with a good personality.

I'm the happiest I have ever been which has improved my personality immensely. This fitness quest enabled my happiness. As you read this book watch the transition of my personality take place. Whereas I initially motivate you with the attention that you get through accomplishments, I later emphasize how motivation can be based on a happy journey of hiking, dating, and experiencing life. I purposely kept the section on compliments and the dark side of my vain attitude as it portrays the person I was at the time. The vain attitude enabled me to become successfully happy yet humble and appreciative. Hence it is an essential part of this book no matter how dark it is.

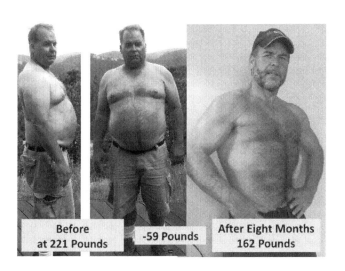

Figure 1 I Lost a Total of 59 Pounds and Toned Up Considerably

1. HOW THIS ALL STARTED

Pretty woman remarking on my physique, "You won't like me because I don't work out.
Me, "I started working out because I didn't like me!"

I lost nearly 60 pounds by not running a single step. Here's how it all started.

One day I just decided I wanted to be fit. I decided I would begin the following Monday. I didn't wait for spring (it was June). I didn't plan on being in shape for the summer. I didn't wait until after the holidays. I didn't seek a certain age at which to begin. I looked in the mirror and decided it was time for me to take control of my health. As it turns out, the mirror became a very valuable asset as I progressed in my effort to become fit.

I had always carried extra weight however I had added an extra 20 pounds as I aged. At age 51 I still had relatively good health yet I was tipping the scales at 231 pounds in January 2013, ten pounds heavier than the weight I was when I started my journey. I was lucky though. I had been diagnosed with high cholesterol my entire life which eventually led to two clogged arteries and a heart attack. We're not talking a cholesterol that crept up from 200 to 220. We're talking a level of 450 with elevated "bad" levels due to a hereditary condition. It is typical for the males in my family to last until about their mid 50's due to this condition. I knew I had to do something if I were to prolong my life.

I had been given a new lease on life by surviving the heart attack with only minor damage. I was under no restrictions from the doctors. As for the clogged arteries, I had grown two new ones around each. Although the new arteries were smaller, they were there and I didn't require a stint.

Surviving the heart attack wasn't my only lucky charm. I had been a daily 2-3 beer social drinker for over 35 years. I had never gotten a DUI yet I knew it was only a matter of time. I liked staying out for live music and did not want to chance a DUI. It was time to quit. I had had a scare in the open Scout that had the top and doors off. I didn't want to push my luck. I have two sons who's future I want to be a part of. I felt that I needed to reduce my drinking if I were to have a future free of the hassles of a DUI. During past weight loss efforts I had learned that drinking was a detriment to my efforts. Therefore, my lifestyle change would definitely assist in curbing drinking. As much as I liked microbrews, it was time to abandon them. Initially I did not stop drinking entirely. Instead, I changed to a lower carb drink. I cover this more in my chapter on alcohol.

I had successfully lost weight on two occasions before in life. During my 20's I had trimmed down to my high school playing weight. In my 30's, I had gotten into a weight loss contest at work and lost 33 ½ pounds in three months and won the contest over the three other guys. Both of those efforts had resulted from diet and exercise, two words I hate. Each time I had starved and cut out fat and meat in my life. I did not cut out bread or beer although I did reduce my drinking considerably. I referred to my past success as S and S for Starve and Sweat. Each time I had suffered with hunger pains and eventually gained the weight back. Those efforts were an example that diets did not work. They were too temporary and hard to maintain.

I knew that this time I had to implement a lifestyle change. I had to establish habits that I would carry with me the rest of my life. Changing eating habits will result in weight loss. I knew I could accelerate the process by also including activities in my lifestyle change. I prefer eating habits and activities over the words diet and exercise. Exercise to me invokes a vision of tedious dedication to unpleasant acts. Instead of exercise, I wanted to participate in fun and rewarding activities that were desirable. Performing the activities outdoors was also a goal. I had spent 30 years in a cubicle and hours in the gym neither of which appealed to me. This time, I was going to do it my way and enjoy the journey. I was going to incorporate fun activities in the outdoors.

In June of 2013 I took photos of myself for reference to gauge my progress against. I then weighed myself and also measured certain areas of my body with a tape measure. I kept track of the gains that I achieved periodically. In the end, I lost 59 pounds, and an inch and a half around my face. I transitioned from a 47 inch waist to a 34 inch waist. My pant size went from spilling over 38" pants down to 30" pants with room to insert three fingers. I lost so much weight that I grew a beard in order to hide the wrinkled skin that became more pronounced on my neck.

It has been over a year since I began and I've successfully kept the weight off. I am much more muscular and my lungs are fully open. No more do I feel any restrictions in them. I use all of their capacity. It is one of the greatest feelings that I can describe. Well, I can almost describe it. You really need to experience it for itself in order to understand the significance.

When I realized I had created a successful, stable lifestyle that kept me fit, I wanted to share my success with others. I had written several books and dozens of technical articles over the years so writing a book was a natural method of sharing my success. I began to investigate the internet and to my surprise, there wasn't a lot of material for men over age 50 on losing weight and shaping up. There was a lot of material for women. I thought that focusing on men over 50 would provide a competitive edge for a book theme and that's how the title was born.

This book is for everyone, not just men over 50. The methods described within apply to any age and both genders. I wish I would have implemented this lifestyle in my 20's or 30's. I recommend that you learn from my experience and implement the change when you can. It took me until I was 51 in order to understand the lifestyle change that led to my success. As I mentioned, I had tried and failed to maintain my weight on two separate occasions. I believe I finally found the key to success and want to share it with you the audience. This third time was a charm as it was the most enjoyable and I was the happiest. This makes me believe I will continue to stay fit as the effort is much easier than the slavery and dedication (not to mention the starvation and injury) that resulted from my prior efforts. Truly this journey has taught me how to enjoy a fit lifestyle. I welcome you to join me and become happy or happier.

In addition to the methods for losing weight that I chose this time, I focus more on the mental aspects and motivation that led to my success. I was miserable during my other weight loss efforts. This time around, I made the effort enjoyable by incorporating fun activities such as dates and visits to the incredible beauty of Colorado into my routine. Instead of being restricted to a gym, I moved my equipment out to the deck and overlooked the Rocky Mountains. Instead of spending money on a club membership and equipment, I saved money on food and by not buying alcohol. My food consumption went down. The foods I chose were more filling and as a result, I ate less. Also, the foods were actually lower in cost as I removed processed foods and replaced them with low carb protein based foods. These foods are actually cheaper overall.

I developed frugal ways to incorporate everyday objects into my routines. As a result, I saved even more money by leveraging that which was around me instead of spending money. I shopped at second hand stores. I took advantage of equipment that friends were throwing away. I used every trick that I could to put a positive spin on this effort. By doing so, it was much more palatable and easier to implement. I made it easy. You can make it easy too. I provide the methods for making your weight loss effort a desirable and rewarding journey.

I set other boundaries that helped keep me motivated. Due to a back injury, I chose not to jar my spine by running. I lost nearly 60 pounds without ever running a single step. Instead, I climbed elevations to increase my aerobic activity.

What surprised me most is how easy it has been to maintain my weight and continue to improve on muscle tone. During my weight loss effort I skipped entire days of activity. I occasionally went outside of my eating habits. Now I can actually skip several days and eat what I want while still keeping fit. I have optimized my maintenance routine in the same manner I optimized my weight loss effort. Note that I started with a restricted menu that I could easily control. Since then, I have introduced foods in increments at a level that allowed me to see their impact on my weight. I still center on low carb proteins. I supplement that mostly with fruits and nuts. One thing I refused to give up was coffee. That did not hinder my success.

Anyone who is reading this book CAN achieve a level of fitness regardless of the state of their health. It really comes down to WANTING to succeed not physical ability. 90% of the effort will be mental. If a person like me who has had a heart attack and is paralyzed can do this, you can. The key is finding the routine that best works for you. I had established the basics for my success due to my previous efforts yet there was still some trial and error that ensued on this journey. Most likely you will also find that only certain things work for you as well. Each routine is different for each person. Knowing this, I provide basic instruction for success instead of a regiment like other books. Just because a particular routine worked for one person doesn't mean it will work for all. Go into this journey realizing that you will have to find your own situation that best fits your abilities and your lifestyle. I provide you with the tools and methods to succeed. You will simply have to adapt these to find your optimal routine.

2. ACCOMPLISHMENTS

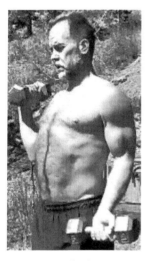

Figure 2 I Liked Working Out on the Deck in the Sunshine. It was 43 Degrees During the Filming of This Sequence

This book wouldn't be complete without listing accomplishments and milestones I passed along the way. The gains and results that I achieved continuously helped drive me to the next level. There was an amazing escalation process that I never envisioned from the beginning losing first 20 pounds, then 30, then 40, then 50, finally 59 pounds. Initially I thought that I would just start with a routine and stick with to maybe get below 200 pounds from 221. I learned so much about my body and more importantly about what works and what doesn't when it comes to shedding weight. As I learned and progressed, I kept losing more and more weight beyond my initial goals. I captured as much of the process as I could in photos and by recording my weight and dimensions. I am presenting this method in a way that you can apply it to your efforts. I'd suggest you also record your progress. It is so easy in this digital era of cameras, applications, and spreadsheets.

The methods for getting to these levels were key to my success. I would set goals and then surpass them. I exceeded goals I never thought possible in the beginning. The progress that I made was due to setting realistic goals and then being patient while I pursued them. Success was due mostly to following through with persistence and motivation; the key differentiators between this and other weight loss books that focus on diet and exercise routines. As with any effort of this nature, the goals were achieved slowly. There were times when I thought my stomach would never go down and of course it crossed my mind that I should just give up because my efforts appeared to be useless; however they weren't. It's has been over a year since I started and the weight is still off. I sport a nice flat stomach and muscular physique that generates a lot of compliments. Nothing is more rewarding than the reaction from those who haven't seen me since my heavier days.

This effort was not without disappointment however realize that I ultimately persevered and you can too. You will mostly realize gains if you persist. Like any effort, you will also recede and hit plateaus. These are a natural part of life. These were actually motivators that pushed me to work harder. The weight didn't go on quickly so don't expect to drop it quickly. Give your body time and it will respond.

I would look at my love handles in the mirror and think I would never lose them. Eventually I lost the love handles and created a torso with ripped abdominal muscles. The fact that my stomach did tone up and the way that it did are probably the most important things that I can tell you. I had always had a pendulous belly that I disliked. Now when I see another that looks like I did, I think, "I can easily transition that to muscle."

I present my results towards the end of this chapter. The beginning of this chapter is where I tell you the phases and changes that I made in order to keep the progress on track. I believe that you will discover the same thing that I did as you pursue your goal; that no one single routine will work for everyone. In fact, the methods that I provide here are suggestions that will lead you to a mental state and a routine that works for you. This is where I believe this book is different than other fitness publications. Instead of dictating a routine and telling you what to do and eat, I help you to discover what works while narrating my success story. I only achieved success through trial and error, not by doing so many repetitions of so many exercises. It is very important that you realize this and discover what works for you rather than trying to implement what worked for me. We are two different people and therefore we will require two different routines. Therefore the "what to do" routines are left to the Appendix while the main body focusses on "how to" succeed. In this work I am telling you how to get motivated and find a successful lifestyle rather than dictating what you should do.

In order to understand my accomplishments you must understand me as a person. By doing so, you will see why I was able to transition my physical condition to a desirable level. The important points for improving my situation include my attitude on life as well as how my schedule allowed me to achieve my milestones. Notice I didn't mention the "exercises" I did. Although I do present the various activities, I again want to emphasize that success is more about mental attitude and planning as well as performing a routine than it is about doing the actual physical workout. We all have a certain amount of time available to dedicate to our workout. The secret lies in how to maximize that time as well as how to MAKE time by stealing from periods in your life that don't yield results. It's called dedication and we are all born with it. It just takes a little effort to initiate it. Initiation is much easier when you realize the incentives that result from the benefits of health and fitness.

As I approached my late 40's and life began to become less affluent from my six figure salaries, an amazing change came over me; the more I lost (possession wise, not weight), the happier I became. I developed a simple philosophy during this time:

I don't have many expectations. Therefore I'm rarely disappointed especially if things don't materialize. If blessings do occur, they become an unexpected gifts.

By not having expectations in the first place, I avoided being disappointed had I not been blessed. Think deeply about this philosophy. Lower your expectations and increase your pursuit of happiness. It will make a huge improvement in your life just like it did in mine. It will set you on a path to happiness. Being happy makes it so much easier to implement a lifestyle change towards being happier.

Gifts enlighten us. Disappointment drags us down. This philosophy was very instrumental to my physical improvements. By not having expectations, I was much more relaxed and less apprehensive about the seemingly insurmountable task I was about to undertake. Sixty pounds is a lot of weight to lose. It was 26 percent of my body weight and the equivalent size of a healthy eight year old. Even twenty or thirty pounds could easily have been viewed as astronomical had I let my mind go there. I didn't over anticipate. I didn't have expectations. Instead I kept working and the weight slowly came off. Progress increased my desire to keep improving. This was in fact, a continuous improvement effort. What started as a desire to look trim has turned into a body sculpting success that has provided me with a look that I only dreamed of having. You too can look better than you ever expected. All it takes is following my advice. Don't start out with a huge goal. Instead, be happy with your progress. It's one of the few times in life I'll advise you to look at the hood ornament instead of the road ahead.

We all have that fear of failure that seems to hold us back. Overwhelming tasks tend to illicit the fear on a grander scale. Writing and editing this book is a perfect example. I would put it off and leave it to the last thing I did instead of the first. Like my fitness effort I invoked an attitude change to get this book out first. The fact that you are reading it means I was successful. Put your fitness first and you will be successful.

I never looked at this journey as overwhelming nor did I look at it as a temporary effort. Instead, I viewed it as a journey that never really has an end. In other words, I understood that being fit meant a lifestyle change that would become permanent. In order to change my lifestyle, I viewed myself as living life on this journey that had no destiny. I wasn't going down the same road, I was taking an entirely new route. I got to enjoy life as it occurred instead of always having to worry about getting to my goal which is the same as worrying about getting to a destination. This is a very important secret for a fit life. Many people lose weight only to gain it back. They work very hard at getting to a goal only to ease up and slip back into a lifestyle that's less structured (notice I didn't say easier as this journey is easy once you get the hang of it). The secret is to live fit all of the time rather than think you can work hard for a period and then slack off. The real secret is to be happy with your routine thus making it much easier to implement and continue to practice. In that way, you will be more likely to keep burning the calories and monitoring your intake. For example, I replaced watching television shows with working out as a way to substitute unproductive time with productive time. I do however offer advice on how to work out and enjoy television. To me, TV is such a waste of time. You accomplish nothing while viewing television. It's made worse by the way programming has gone from informative documentaries to profiling the lives of idiots in reality shows. The same goes for unproductive time spent socializing by texting and using the computer. Limit the unproductive time. Schedule time to invest in your body as well as your health rather than wasting time on meaningless tasks. Make your tasks enjoyable doing activities such as hiking, walking, climbing stairs, or playing with children. Think of you, your image to others, your health, and your family. Do you want to end up in a hospital bed and helpless? Where would you rather die, outdoors or in a care facility that reeks of urine being attended to by people you don't know? The choice is yours, decide now. Start your journey and control your destination. Being fit will help to avoid debilitating diseases and will prolong your life. It can also be fun so choose activities that you enjoy while burning fat. Again, enjoy the journey without worrying about a destination.

As I said, you accomplish nothing while watch TV. So change the situation. Accomplish *something* while you are watching TV. When I did want to watch the occasional sports event on TV, I made sure I did it with the weights and dumb bells present. Keep your dumbbells and a mat in the TV room. Leaving them squirreled away in a room you never enter means you are less likely to use them. I earned my right to watch TV and accomplished something while doing so. As it turns out, the exercise made for a great distraction from commercials.

There was a period where I was so busy that I didn't watch TV. When I did return to viewing television, I realized some things. The number one thing is that TV commercials can cause you to overeat. I found myself watching the commercials and craving the food that was advertised. So how does one circumvent the urge? My success came by working out during the commercials. Do something to direct your focus away from the commercials. Mute the TV to avoid the distraction of the sound. Listen to music instead. Have a music source available that is loaded with songs you want to hear. Keeping your music loaded smart phone and some ear buds nearby helps you to focus on something other than commercials.

I'll reveal another secret here. Watching TV usually takes place in a relaxing, restful position such as in a chair, on a couch, or in a bed. I realized that keeping my rest periods to the eight hour block of time that I slept while replacing the times I was awake with periods of exercise actually gave me more energy and reduced fatigue. I felt better too. So if you're going to watch TV, get something out of it. Exercise as you watch and at least accomplish something instead of wasting time doing nothing. You only need a certain amount of restful sleep a day. Don't waste your time or your body lying around watching TV or doing other sedentary dead end efforts. Instead, get the blood pumping by activating your heart, lungs, and muscles. Try these methods to see if they work for you as well as they did for me. At the very least, you will begin to start feeling better and sleeping more effectively. My 28 year old housemate said he was popping out of bed versus resetting the alarm after only a couple of sessions of exercise. Simply put, these recommendations work.

There are however two aspects to a fitness efforts, the loss phase and the maintenance phase. What is amazing about my accomplishment is that I enjoy my routine so much that I still do the efforts I did to lose this weight even though I am pretty much have hit a plateau and I am in a maintenance mode. The key takeaway is: I made my loss effort a routine that was so enjoyable, I still do it. In fact I crave it. I want to emphasize that this can be a fun journey rather than a painful, tedious process. It is also very rewarding as you begin to see that sculpted body emerge in the mirror and start receiving compliments. Two benefits already have surfaced (having fun and rewarding) and we haven't even considered the fact that a healthier you will also result from these efforts. I address the loss and maintenance aspects more in the phases discussion at the end of the chapter. For now just realize that my attitude from the beginning helped me make the lifestyle change and stick to it. It has now been over a year and I've kept the weight off and toned considerably.

My current philosophy now that I am in my 50's is a very different approach to life than my earlier years as a type A driven person. I accomplished many things by driving myself extremely hard during my 20's and 30's. I was rarely happy during that time as I always wanted more instead of being satisfied with what I had. I never seemed to reach my goals and if I did, they didn't satisfy me. I was impatient and grouchy if not greedy. In a nutshell, I was expecting too much of myself and life in a manner where I was experiencing a lot of disappointment while receiving virtually no gifts. I had expectations which meant I was often experiencing disappointment when the expectations were not met. What a change that has come over me since I eliminated expectations. By not over expecting, I've now made it very easy on myself to meet and exceed goals. By adopting my attitude, you too can meet your goals while experiencing pleasure rather than pain. Take this attitude seriously. Don't expect anything from your efforts. Instead, put the emphasis on enjoying the process. The benefits will come as unexpected gifts when you see the results of your progress. For you the younger crowd, think twice about this. Did you ever notice how your grandparents seem less stressed and more appreciative of little things? That used to drive me nuts that older people settled for less and had lackluster goals. Call it geezing or whatever but these methods are best adopted early in life if you are to achieve happiness. Take it from someone who learned the hard way. I didn't take the blinders off until reality slapped me in the face.

My drive in those early years did pay off with success, I'll admit that. I was the first one to obtain a Master's Degree on either side of my immediate family. I was also the first to get an engineering degree from a university (although a cousin did get one from a trade school). Once I achieved my education, I vigorously pursued success in the corporate world. I was climbing at a pace that I wasn't happy with so I looked for a small business as a method to excel faster. I always wanted to be in a position to retire early by creating a product or business that would elevate my income faster than my career was. I wanted to have enough capital built up so that work would be optional. I moved my retirement ages from 30 to 35 to 40 to 45 to 50 and here I sit writing this book and unable to retire at age 52. I finally came to realize that I had expectations that were unreasonable. I wasn't living life in the present, I was fretting it away by hoping for the future that wasn't possible nor was it achievable in the manner I was operating in. I knew I had to change my outlook on life if I were to succeed. When I relaxed, I became happier and was able to focus first on my body and then on writing this book. Who knows what is next? It could be the golden ticket to retirement or it could make me happier by sharing my success and enabling another.

One key fact that keeps me going on my current routine is that I enjoy life along the way. Two of my aerobic routines are done outdoors in the beauty of Colorado. These routines are climbing a steep trail on the side of Bergen Mountain and climbing the stairs at Red Rocks Amphitheatre. Each offers twenty minutes of aerobic, lung expanding exercise. More importantly, I never tire of the beauty and the atmosphere of my routines. I'm not stuck inside on some boring treadmill. Even if I were, I'd adjust my environment to be pleasant. It could be as simple as adding music and pleasing visual enhancements such as paintings, pictures, or scenery scrolling on a computer or TV screen. I can adjust my environment and do so as an incentive to keep going. With all of the media devices available to us these days, it is easy to bring visual benefits into a gym or club too. Although those days of working inside a club are long gone for me as I prefer to be outdoors and perform my routine at home, I encourage you to do whatever works best for you. If it's a gym or club membership, then do it. If it is performing outside activities then do it. I became aware of the awesome place I live and the many opportunities that existed right outside my door. You can too. It's as simple as rowing a pond or skating on it rather than driving by it every day without taking advantage of the benefits that it offers.

I also adjust my life to the weather. I work inside when the weather is uncooperative and exercise outdoors when the weather permits. This provides two important methods for staying on my routine. First, I limit my excuses by taking advantage of the nice weather when it is present. I know I must do it now before the bad weather moves in. Second, I plan my workout as a part of my routine rather than it being an afterthought that gets pushed out and eliminated due to poor planning. In the area of Colorado where I live; summer days have sunny mornings while rain moves in during the afternoon. Therefore I do an outdoor activity in the morning and work inside in the afternoon.

Writing provides a lifestyle that allows me to share my success as well as implement my lifestyle change. Writing has been a part of my life for several decades. I am telling you this because it is important how my vocational lifestyle includes other aspects that make my fit lifestyle work for me. In my mid 30's I had written a book. It was a trail guide titled, "The Four Wheel Drive Trails of Arizona." I had turned my hobby into a successful business. Writing a book is a great way to generate cash. Once you have completed it, you can pretty much sit back and collect the income. Unlike the situation I faced when I published back in 1996, nowadays one can avoid printing costs by going directly to an ebook which is nothing more than a computer file with the book text and figures. In other words, I don't have to gamble on a large printing investment not paying off with this book like I did with my first one. Although I didn't make enough off of my first book to retire, there was a great happiness that I could enjoy my hobby and profit from it. I took this same happiness in my weight loss effort and decided to share it with you. I hope it puts you on the road to success. I also hope you find a way to profit from your interests like I once did.

Writing a book can be very profitable and rewarding as you share your story and incentivize others. This paragraph gets back to how attitude relates to life. By sharing my journey with you, I'm once again attempting to profit from my "hobby" of daily exercise. I however have no expectations for a monetary return on this investment. I will do my best to share my success in hopes that you too can improve your life and pass the success along to others. Your success will be reward enough. Creating one successful story will be reward enough. I have already inspired some of my Facebook family to begin their fitness journeys. I am expanding to encourage others via this book as well as via social media such as a website, blog, youtube videos, as well as websites such as LinkedIn and Twitter. That is my goal in writing this book, creating success stories like my own while expanding my possibility of being successful. After all you are reading this book because you want results. How can I share my success if I don't succeed myself? Remember, you're on a journey here that is mental. My incentive to share my success helps maintain my lifestyle from a mental standpoint which keeps me on my physical journey.

Writing a best seller is very difficult so I'm not expecting this book to be a success. In that manner, any success it does experience will be an unexpected gift rather than a disappointment due to not meeting expectations. Like my weight loss effort, I don't have any expectations in terms of sales. I'm enjoying writing it and filling a market niche oh "How to" lose weight rather than "what to do" to lose weight. I am enjoying sharing my journey. I hope you are enjoying reading about it and see the value of implementing the methods that led to my success. They can be applied in many areas of life besides fitness and weight loss.

During my market research for this book I learned a lot about the fitness craze and how commercial it is. Like anything else, fitness is a business. College is an example of a business. Nobody gives a hoot about your education with the exception of maybe the dedicated educators. The universities and schools are in it for the cash. The same goes with fitness. Find one person that isn't endorsing something such as themselves, a supplement, or a program that you pay for. You can't. I'm writing this book to prove that an average Joe can successfully implement weight loss without investing a lot of money. I also aim to prove that the average Joe can share his success without commercial backing. If you like this book, please recommend it and support my effort to live the American dream.

In my earlier weight loss efforts, I had confined myself to a gym where all exercises other than jogging were performed indoors. Being a lover of the outdoors, I was determined that this weight loss effort would be accomplished outdoors where I was happier and more likely to continue my efforts. In a manner similar to potentially creating income from my hobby, I was positioning myself to be happy while losing weight by enjoying the outdoors. I was combining accomplishment with something I enjoyed doing. I also enjoy writing so the benefits were two fold, I got fit and wrote my story. Again, mindset and mental attitude adjustments such as this will give you a much better chance at success. I admittedly experience pain and fatigue during workouts as will you. It's just a part of the process. Overall I feel awesome much more than I experience displeasure. I did my best to minimize the more unpleasant times by focusing more on high repetitions at lighter weights than progressing in the amount of weight. However, I feel so good after working out, these moments of unpleasantness are worth it. Some of the exercises did produce pain however it was a "good hurt". In other words, there is a certain taxation of your body that results in the generation of endorphins that make you feel good. Runners will tell you this as they experience a "runners high" where they almost feel like they are floating. For the most part, I enjoy my workout. There are certain exercises that I enjoy more than others yet I know having a well proportioned physique requires that I hit all of the major muscle groups evenly. Some of the more challenging and taxing exercises may fatigue me more than others. I just do as many repetitions as I can and then do as many sets as I can to get to my goal of 50 total reps per routine. I gut through it like my mentors Vince Lombardi and Bart Starr did. I get joy out of challenging myself and succeeding. As I tell my sons, if it were easy, everyone will be doing it. Now is your chance to stand out in a crowd of those who take the easy route.

I can't say if my more relaxed philosophy of my current way of thinking would have resulted in my success to a level that driving myself so hard did in my 20's and 30's. I can however say this, I wasn't happy back then and I'm much happier now. I am enjoying the journey and have implemented it as a lifestyle change. I'm less concerned with the destination than I am with enjoying life in the present. Patience is a learned trait which I employ now and should have had more of in my younger years. The quicker you learn patience, the happier you will become and more importantly, the easier it will be to attain your desired level of fitness. I had been told that patience resulted in happiness time and time again yet I had to experience it for myself. For you younger readers, take note; be patient. Implement the changes now. I wish I had implemented them at an earlier age.

There is an old saying that has relevance here, "Rome wasn't built in a day." Rome was a successful city in one of the most propsperous civilizations of all time yet it took years to get there. For all of you reading this book my experiences taught me to be patient and patience is what weight loss is all about. If you think about your additional weight, you didn't put it on in a week so don't expect it to come off in a week.

Remember, this is a book about mental ability more so than physical gain. Learning and applying patience is a mental effort, not a physical one. Mental effort is the key to success. It will drive the physical effort. You will be amazed at how much mental focus will turn physical efforts from exhausting to rewarding.

It was essential to spell out my attitude in order to fully understand how my accomplishments where obtained and milestones surpassed. When I first started this effort, I weighed 221 pounds. My initial goal was to weigh less than 200 pounds. I had lost a similar amount about ten years earlier mostly by walking and swimming and partially implementing a low carb diet. This was actually a fourth effort of less proportion as I bottomed out at 200 pounds rather than somewhere in the 160's range that my physique is most desirable. It seems as though I go through this every decade. This loss of ten pounds in my forties was not as impactful as the two efforts where I lost more in my 20's and 30's. My kids often referred to that period in my forties by commenting about how good I looked back then. On previous tries at weight loss, I had dropped 30 pounds per each of the two efforts getting down to 159 pounds and around 160 at age 25 and age 32 respectively. However my children were not around to see those efforts. Still, a loss of ten pounds in my forties and the fact that my kids remembered it is worth mentioning. Remember that incentive plays a big part in achieving success. The incentive of positive feedback by my kids helped drive me to again seeking fitness. I want them to be proud of their dad. I don't think that being lazy and fat made them proud. I represent an example for these two, fine young man. If that example is a fit figure versus a decrepit old man, I am incentivized by their pride in me.

Incidentally, I pushed myself too hard during that last weight loss effort in my thirties and wound up slightly but permanently paralyzed in my right leg due to rupturing a disk in my back. The injury was initialized during the first weight loss effort in my 20's. I was going about it all wrong in my earlier years. I was pushing too hard and exercising incorrectly which resulted in a permanent injury. Back then I always had to progress higher in weight and get bigger. I pushed my body beyond its limits and it finally resulted in an injury. I had ruptured a disk to a point where the gel inside the fibrous disk caused the disk to protrude against a nerve that ran through the spinal column. This in turn cut off the signals to my right leg resulting in a partial paralysis. The pain from this type of an injury is almost unbearable. I'd suggest taking precautions to avoid it.

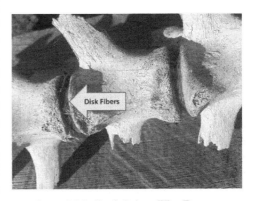

Figure 3 My Back Injury Was Due to a Ruptured Disk

In this book, I share from my past experience that caused my injury. I take a slower, more methodical pace. I have successfully been on my routine with no damage to my back. In fact, for the few times it did bother me during this effort, I discovered ways to loosen it up and stop the pain. I took precautions such as wearing a weight belt I bought for three dollars at a second hand store. I used lower amounts of dumb bell weight and increased by repetitions. Once my strength began to improve and my weight in body fat lessened, I began using heavier weights to replace the fat with muscle. Still, I took it slower than the early days by using weights I could manage rather than weights that taxed my ligaments, tendons, bones, and spine. I noticed that my muscles and bones can still handle the weight however my tendons seem to suffer now that I'm above 50. I adapted to my limitations. I'd suggest you do that as well.

As a result of this history of weight loss, I expected to drop maybe twenty to thirty pounds when I started again at age 51 in

June 2013. I felt that being under 200 pounds would be quite an achievement as losing weight is as difficult for me as it is for anyone. I had been chunky the majority of my life so for me, carrying extra weight was a lifestyle. I felt that 185 pounds was my optimal weight however at a net loss of 36 pounds from my starting point of 221, it was a goal that appeared far beyond reach. Never in my mind did I believe that I would lose nearly 60 pounds and be extremely close to a six pack set of abdominal muscles while weighing under 165 pounds. For the month of February 15, 2014 to March 18, 2014 I've fluctuated between 55 and 59 pounds lost (166 and 162 pounds total weight down from my 221 starting weight). I can't seem to get to sixty pounds or the illusive six pack….although I believe shaving the Yeti might show six pack definition in my abdominals. While editing this book by creating the still shots from videos, I did see the six pack rips in various poses. Still, a six pack is not visible when I am in a static, rest pose. In a way this is good because I always have two goals, sixty pounds lost and six pack abs. If I'm always pursuing them, I'm always maintaining if not losing. It's very strange how setting a goal I never achieve keeps me motivated. This goal of sixty pounds and a six pack keeps me motivated now that I'm close. I compare it to a dog chasing a car. What is the dog going to do with the car when he catches it? The fun is in the chase. That way 60 pounds and six pack abs don't become an expectation that disappoints me should I not achieve them. Instead, I'm focusing on the journey rather than the destination in much the same manner as a dog enjoying the chase. This is a key mental method that helps one become successful. Enjoy the journey and don't worry about the destination. The ultimate destination in life is death. I hope that helps you to understand my philosophy better.

Had I set a goal this large (60 pounds of eventual loss) in the beginning, I would never have gotten to the level I had. Again, the journey and the milestones are what made this possible. As I surpassed goals, I kept setting new ones, 20, then 30, then 40, then 50 pounds. Don't look too far ahead or set expectations; especially unreasonable ones. Live for the present and celebrate your success to date. Make your routine and eating habits an enjoyable lifestyle and stick to them. Pursue activities that make you happy. Don't suffer now for results later. Enjoy the journey as life was meant to be lived in the present. Memories give us nostalgic happiness of the past. The future is based on expectations which can disappoint. This perspective works for me. I don't have expectations therefore I'm rarely disappointed. I can't emphasize that enough.

Now that I have established my initial goals and my attitude on life, it's time to show how this amazing transition took place. I look at the milestones and think about what I accomplished and I still can't believe I did it. Again, it took patience and appreciation for the gifts that presented themselves along the way. I knew the weight would come off if I stuck to the eating habits and lifestyle change (again, I don't like the words diet and exercise). The amount of success that I had is the reason I wrote this book. I want others to experience these accomplishments as well so I chose to share them with you, the audience. More importantly, please consider implementing a lifestyle change that will make you happier.

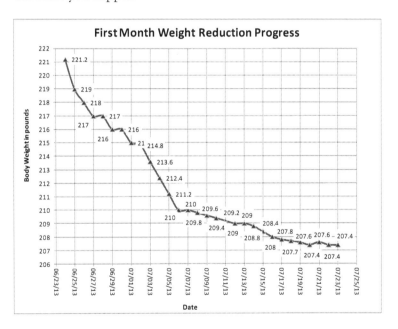

Figure 4 First Month Weight Loss Progress

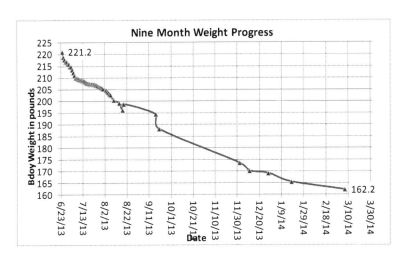

Figure 5 Nine Month Weight Loss Progress (Body Weight)

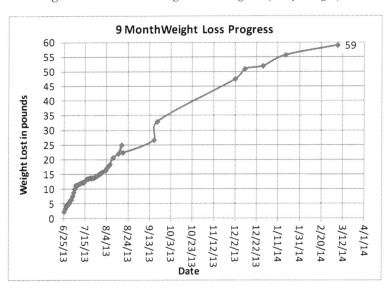

Figure 6 Nine Month Weight Loss Progress (Pounds Lost)

Table 1 Progress in Areas of the Body I Chose to Monitor

			06/24/13	12/2/2013
weight	lbs	weight	221.2	173 2/3
face	in	length	22	20 3/4
waist	in	length	47	37
lower waist	in	length	42	36
bicep	in	length	16	13 3/4
chest				41 3/4

Without further delay, here's the list of accomplishments as they occurred. After the table, I'll summarize everything that combines my attitude and the milestones/accomplishments.

Table 2 List of Accomplishments

Accomplishment/ Comment/Milestone	Date	Elapsed Time (months)	Body Weight (pounds)
Started working out at age 51. Weighed 221 pounds. 47" waist	Sunday June 25, 2013	0	221.2
Lost 7 pounds the 1st week; 9 pounds by July 6	July 6, 2013	0.5	210
Down 14 pounds	July 23, 2013	1.0	207.4

Table 2. List of Accomplishments (continued)

Accomplishment/ Comment/Milestone	Date	Elapsed Time (months)	Body Weight (pounds)
August Golden Car Cruise	August 3, 2013	1.2	204.8
Down 22 pounds….	August 18, 2013	1.8	196.2
Told that my liver would shrink eventually	Nurse friend told me in late August	1.8	
Your shoulders have good definition	Comment from friend on Vail trip the week before Labor Day weekend	2.2	
Down 25 pounds	Labor Day weekend 2013	2.2	

Table 2. List of Accomplishments (continued)

Accomplishment/ Comment/Milestone	Date	Elapsed Time (months)	Body Weight (pounds)
Gained some weight back eating party food and drinking alcohol	Labor Day	2.2	Didn't record
Down 35 pounds; told I was fat on Facebook yet told I looked like Jack LaLane by a close friend	October 2	3.2	185.2
Friend slaps me on shoulder, remarks on physique and inquires as to whether I've been working out	Mid October	3.4	
I stopped drinking entirely; eventually dropped 25 more pounds	October 26, 2013	4	
A waiter where I get the weekly ribs special remarks how I look "cut" in a medium sized Tshirt. Within a month I'm wearing smalls.	November 2013	5	

Table 2. List of Accomplishments (continued)

Accomplishment/ Comment/Milestone	Date	Elapsed Time (months)	Body Weight (pounds)
Hit 40 pounds lost	November 25, 2013	4.5	
Bought 32" jeans; picked up some with a 30" waist mistaking it for 30" inseam. The 30's fit! Surprise! Surprise!	Week of Thanksgiving	5	
I noticed my abdominals caved in and felt like I finally had tight abs	First week of December 2013 after two weeks on Pilates power machine	5.2	173.7
Ex girlfriend (dated Sept 11 – Nov 23) sees me after a month. First words out of her mouth were, "You look good."	December 20, 2013	6	170.2

Table 2. List of Accomplishments (continued)

Accomplishment/ Comment/Milestone	Date	Elapsed Time (months)	Body Weight (pounds)
Comparison photo 52 pounds lost	December 28, 2013	6	169.2
Friend remarks on sharp edge of my rib cage protruding (it used to be my stomach that protruded)	Arizona visit January 1, 2014	6.2	

Table 2. List of Accomplishments (continued)

Accomplishment/ Comment/Milestone	Date	Elapsed Time (months)	Body Weight (pounds)
Hit 53 pounds lost 	February 2013	7	164
Hit 59 pounds lost, grew a beard to hide the wrinkles that resulted in my neck 	March 7, 2013	8	162.2

I feel that sharing this journey with you is the best way to incentivize you to start your new and exciting fit lifestyle. As you can see, I have a story to tell about my accomplishments and achieving milestones. The story ended in success. There is no better proof that something works than success. There is a very important point to be made about these accomplishments. They were achieved through consistency in food consumption and by changing my activity routine in various phases. I purposely don't use the words, "diet and exercise" as they seem so temporary.

Consistency of consumption means that I pretty much ate the same group of foods throughout the entire effort. The initial emphasis on was low carb and high protein. I avoided wheat based products. If it was white (bread, flour based, rice), I didn't eat it. The exception was cheese which is low in carbs. I avoided milk as it has carbs. I can only remember two days where I felt famished. In my previous efforts I had hunger pains and headaches due to my menu of choice during those times and my effort to starve the weight off. This time my intake consisted of eggs and bacon in the morning, cheese sticks, and meat such as chicken and fish. I would have chicken wings on Sundays and get $1.25 per ribs on Tuesday at a local restaurant that had a weekly special. I could get three meals out of ten, "dry" (no sauce) ribs. At about four dollar per meal, I was eating well for a decent price. I usually had wings left over from Sunday and could have them for a second meal. I would cook fish or chicken in quantities and heat them up through the week. I liked Salmon mostly as it is one of my favorites. At first I ate just baked Salmon. As I progressed I introduced Salmon patties which I used eggs and meatloaf or Lipton Onion soup seasoning in (although both contained carbs). The introduction of salmon patties took place well into the 40 pound loss time frame as I was more in a maintenance mode than a loss mode at that point.

As my weight loss attained goals beyond which I ever thought possible, I still was frustrated with the lack of hitting 60 pounds and getting to a six pack. I resorted to the internet and learned that a six pack is more a function of body fat than it is of improving abdominal muscles. This rang true with me as I was doing upwards of 1500 reps per day on my abdominals alone yet I never seemed to get ripped. Once I learned that intake was the dominate factor over exercise, I went to egg whites only, cut out the bacon, and introduced broccoli and tuna fish as my meat sources. That level of restriction of foods became too much so I eased back a bit. It was overwhelming me to have set an expectation of achieving six pack abs. I had strayed from my philosophy of enjoying the journey and instead had set an expectation. This resulted in disappointment. I abandoned my quest for six pack abs. The result was I was much happier with my lifestyle as well as my looks. I didn't want the stringy muscle look that was resulting due to the loss of body fat. I preferred the smoother look with some fat. To me, that's a healthier look. Note that this is a perfect example of the continued reference to trial and error. I give something about three weeks and if it doesn't work, I continue to change until I find something that does produce the desired results. I had restricted my eating habits to an area that was uncomfortable. This would have destroyed my lifestyle. I went back to a happier place of viewing occasional glimpses of a six pack versus having a predominant constant one.

Eventually I began to introduce healthy foods (beyond pure protein) that contained simple sugars such as fruits. I avoided complex sugars. I focused on natural foods while avoiding preservative infested processed foods. I also noticed my legs were cramping quite a bit so I started to eat a daily banana for more potassium to offset the cramping. I started eating an orange per day in order to introduce simple sugars for energy and carb absorption. My downfall was nuts. They are ok at two handfuls a day however I was eating up to a jar a day. Although I was doing upwards of 300 sit ups per day, it was too cold to do my aerobic mountain climb up Bergen Mountain or stair climb at Red Rocks. I was taking in calories and not burning them. I cut out the nuts and regained my aerobic activity of about two sessions every three days. This period was a learning process in consumption of what worked and what didn't. Granted I was in the latter stages of loss where those last few pounds come off very slowly. Reintroducing the carbs in nuts stalled my effort. I now eat nuts regularly and don't seem to gain anything. They curb my appetite, don't require refrigeration, and are portable. I keep nuts in my vehicle and bedroom for quick snacks. Occasionally a raccoon gets in the open Scout when the top is off and eats them. I've learned to take them in at night.

Note that having food prepared or ready as leftovers means that you have items in place which meet your diet requirements. When you have to scramble and prepare a meal, you're more likely to eat out of convenience and cheat outside your chosen area of foods that result in weight loss progress. Pick foods that are convenient or prepare foods in advance so that you reduce the tendency to cheat and avoid instant gratification.

So that's the consumption part. I'm not a doctor nor am I a nutritionist. If I were to evaluate my success it would be broken down into a simple summary whereas I lost weight by using my stored fat as energy that I normally ingested as carbohydrates. By having a protein based menu that limited carb intake, I was able to tone and build muscle that provided a good use of the protein I ingested. As a man with high cholesterol, I was successful on an Atkins based diet. Although some doctors may not agree with my philosophy, you can't argue with success.

The real losses (and muscle definition gains) are attributed to the phases of change in my activity routine. Theses phases are presented in a table as well as in text that relates them to the storyline of this effort. The phase story can be summarized as being two part: improvements in weight lifting and increasing aerobic activity.

I started out with small 15 pound dumbbells and 50 reps each for various muscles in my chest, shoulders, and back. Gradually, I increased to 100 reps. By December (6 months in) I lost a lot of weight (52 pounds) using this routine however I was lanky. I wanted to be bulkier and have more muscle size as well as definition. I knew the way to do it was to increase the size of the weights. I kept my eye on Craigslist and when a pair of 45 pound dumb bells became available, I snagged them up. They were so heavy at first that I could barely walk up a small hill to my car with them. Initially, it would take all I had to swing them up in place for bench presses. As time has progressed, I can now move them fairly easily. They still challenge me at certain times with certain movements however I can get upwards of 30 reps on the incline bench and reps in shrugs and side bends making them an optimal overall weight for me. I listen to my body and use lower 25 pound weights for exercises that tax my ligaments and limits. My success was realized by focusing on 50 reps per routine versus increase dumb bell weight. Make a similar adjustment and you will succeed. This will help you avoid injury or quitting due to attempting something that is overly difficult.

I did injure my left bicep tendon due to the excessive weight of the heavier 45 pound dumb bells. The sideways force was the cause of the problem. I have since rehabilitated the tendon and now take special care when moving the weights into position for my bench presses. I also had created a slight injury in my left shoulder. Once I started doing shoulder shrugs properly this injury subsided. It did result in me favoring my right side. I noticed this in some of the still shots and videos that were the source for the figures in the Appendix. Note that working out in a mirror helps you to realize and correct for these imbalances in your movements. As vain as it may seem, having a mirror available can help you correct your movements before they cause or enhance an injury.

Aerobic activity for optimal weight loss is best described in one word; elevation. When I was walking on flat ground, I wasn't losing weight nor was I gaining lung capacity. Running was out of the question as I didn't want to jar my back and aggravate my already damaged disk. Swimming was out due to the expense and time involved to go to the pool, change, swim, and shower. I had to find something that would elevate my breathing and heart rate. When I went on a group hike in July 2013 at Red Rocks to observe the moonrise over Denver, I was hyperventilating and dragging along at the back of the pack. Shortly afterwards, my friend Wilhelmina invited me to hike Bergen Mountain with her guests that were attending a weight loss boot camp. Again the elevation was taxing and pushing my breathing to a high and uncomfortable level. It was at that point I realized the value of climbing an elevation in terms of a weight burning, lung expanding aerobic activity. As it turned out, the hike to a certain overlook was perfect and it was right outside my door. It gained 500 feet in elevation over 1.2 miles and at my best, took me 25 minutes to traverse. For the most part, it went up an elevated grade with a varying slope. It took me three months of trying in order to complete this hike without stopping to catch my breath. There were challenges along the way such as snow and the time I got caught in a serious lightning storm. The lightening was hitting on either side of me while the rain poured down in torrents. I thought for sure I was a goner sticking out on the mountainside like I was. I kept preparing to hit the ground if I felt my hair start to tingle indicating a strike was inbound. I always carried a lug wrench, walking stick, or ski poles in case I encountered a cougar on Bergen Mountain. And of course, I had my camera phone along to document the journey or call for help if necessary. The phone also had music on it that inspired me. Occasionally the snow would be deep enough to slow me down. I did turn back due to snow on a couple of occasions however I never needed snow shoes. For your convenience I have enclosed some pictures of my overlook hike. As you can see from the stunning beauty and views, it wasn't difficult to incentivize myself to hike every day.

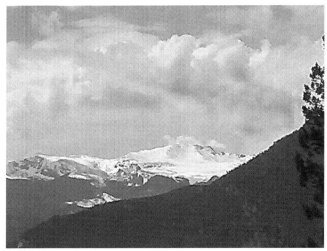
Figure 7 This View of Mount Evans to the West Is the Reward That
Awaits Me at the Top of My Climb

About two months into this journey I started dating a girl
who lived down near Denver. I lived about 20 miles away in the
Rocky Mountains in a town called Evergreen. Red Rocks park
was half way between us in Morrison, Colorado. We began to
meet at Red Rocks where I would climb the amphitheater stairs
as a part of my elevation activity. I now climb the stairs four
times per visit. I try to visit two to three times per week. I have
made a pact with myself that I cannot go down the hill without a
stop at Red Rocks. Sometimes this takes up to two hours. I
often get kicked out of the park in the summer as they prepare
for evening activities such as concerts and movies. In the winter,
I face icy stairs and winds. There are no excuses. All of these
inhibitors are anticipated, dealt with, and overcome. I am a
disciple of Vince Lombardi, one of the most successful coaches
of all time. His methods make me successful by finding the drive
within me. As Americans, it is within all of us. Otherwise, we'd
be American'ts.

Climbing Red Rocks amphitheater is a great activity. When
the stairs become too taxing, I walk along the rows of seats while
taking in the view of the rocks or the Denver skyline out on the
Great Plains. When I get my breathing back under control, I
continue my climb. Each time I push a little harder. This has
resulted in my ability to climb the whole venue without stopping.
I used Red Rocks to balance the strength in my legs and offset
the paralysis in my right leg. When doing the benches at Red

Rocks I do ten benches with my right leg to three with my left leg. This roughly three to one ratio has balanced the strength and made up for the lack of nerve control in my right leg due to my paralysis.

I have incorporated other exercises into my Red Rocks visits

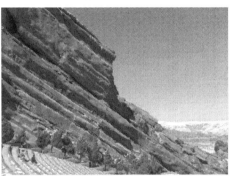

that you can see in the Appendix. In addition to elevation climbs, I'm now hiking a lot with my recent female companion. Again, by incorporating fun and interesting activities into your lifestyle change you will lose at a faster rate and be more likely to stick with it.

Figure 8 I Regularly Climb the Stairs at Red Rocks to Keep My Aerobic Stamina Up

I don't emphasize a workout buddy in this book however they are essential to a lot of people. I do have several buddies that I contact however I'm always prepared to go it alone. I've found workout buddies are unreliable most of the time. I take advantage of them when they are available however I don't let their absence or the disappointment of cancellation deter me. I plan to proceed without them yet enjoy the gift of their presence. I don't have the expectation that they will show up so I don't have the disappointment when they fail to appear. My philosophy again results in success and happiness.

I have optimized my routine for the area I live in. These methods that I preach can be applied by anyone living anywhere. I've expanded and added to my areas where I perform aerobic activities by keeping aware and observing my surroundings for the opportunities that arise. I've done this near my home as well as when I'm travelling. If I can keep going anywhere, you can. I have lived in various parts of the United States and always had my special places like Red Rocks and Bergen Mountain. I would suggest you find your special place that you enjoy and incorporate activities into your visits and travels. If you don't live near an elevation or hill that is a good climb, find a staircase. Use an indoors one during periods of bad weather and an outdoor one such as a high school football field bleachers for nice days. Look for other areas to do dips and upper body exercises such as curls.

In the following table, I present my routine and how it changed as I progressed. My overall goal was to shed the weight and then put weight back on as muscle. This routine worked out quite well for me. It will make a nice guideline for you however because we are different people, it may not be optimal. The key takeaway here is to view the way in which I was able to find a routine and set of activities that worked. The main difference between this book and others is that I show you the activities that worked rather than overwhelming you with an exercise routine that hits every part of the body. The quickest path to failure is to overwhelm yourself. Instead, try routines and optimize your activity so that you are losing weight while enjoying the journey. Start slow like I did using lighter weights and reduced repetitions. Expand to a combination that maintains your desired level of fitness. Optimization comes through a series of trial and error. The phases I present here are a profile of this process. Learn from the process and incorporate it into your routine. By doing so, you will have a better chance at succeeding.

I have saved the detailed description of my routines for the Appendix where they belong as a reference rather than putting them into the main body. They are not in the main body of the book because this book is a "how to" presentation for improving your fitness level and thus saves the "what to" do part for getting fit for reference only.

Table 3 Phases and Routines that Worked for Me

Phase Routine	Period	Elapsed Time (months)	Comments
Aerobic Exercise was walking 1.2 miles around Evergreen Lake	June-July 2013	1	50 foot elevation change wasn't effective for increasing lung capacity
50 reps with 15 pound dumbbells (all groups chest/back/shoulders)	June 23, 2013- August 2013	2	High reps, low weight helped burn carbs
Increased Ab exercises to doing bicycles and boxer twists	July 2013 – March 2013	8	Increased core strength; eventually dropped boxer moves due to being ineffective
Started Climbing Bergen Mountain	July 23 – present	Ongoing	Lungs began expanding, got further every day without stopping
Moved to 100 reps on dumb bells; Broke the routine into two muscle groups (chest and then back/shoulders)	August 2013 – November 2013	3	Higher reps due to hitting plateau with 50 reps
Started climbing Red Rocks	September 2013- present	ongoing	Stairs really made a difference

Table 3 Phases and Routines that Worked for Me (continued)

Phase Routine	Period	Elapsed Time (months)	Comments
Finally made all 1.2 miles of Bergen Mountain without stopping	October 2013	Ongoing	It took a 3 months!
Increased dumbbell weight from 15 to 20 pounds; started doing muscles in 3 groups at a group per day (chest/shoulders/back)	November 2013 – December 2013	2	Started building muscle instead of burning fat
Got a used Pilates Machine	Last week of November		
Started doing side twists on Pilates Machine	November 26 thru December 6, 2013	0.5	Caved in sides of stomach within two weeks
Started doing benches (longer stride) at Red Rocks; 3 on left side, 10 on right due to paralysis in right leg	November 2013 - present	Ongoing	Strength and balance have improved
Started using Pilates Machine as an incline bench	December 6, 2013 to present	ongoing	Started going from lanky to bulky
Started using Pilates Machine for rowing, side pulls, and lat pulls in back	December 6, 2013 to present	ongoing	Improved definition in my back

Table 3 Phases and Routines that Worked for Me (continued)

Phase Routine	Period	Elapsed Time (months)	Comments
Introduced sit ups and leg lifts	December 6, 2013 – present	ongoing	Couldn't do 8 situps at the start; did 500 in February 2014
Found 45 dumb bells on Craigslist;	December 27, 2013 - present	ongoing	Shoulder, chest, and arm size have all improved
Started doing dips at Red Rocks	January 6, 2014 - present	ongoing	Chest size has increased and rounded pectorals nicely
Started doing curls at Red Rocks	February 2014- present	Ongoing	Offset numbness in arms from dips; improved definition of biceps
Started 100 side stretches with 45 pound dumb bells	March, 2014 - present	Ongoing	Final move to remove love handles
Used two 45 pound dumb bells during situps	April 2014	1	Too much strain on arm joints; reduced weight and increased reps
Using 45 pound dumb bell to do 100 sit ups	April 2014 – present	ongoing	Easier on joints and tendons

Table 3 Phases and Routines that Worked for Me (continued)

Phase Routine	Period	Elapsed Time (months)	Comments
Noticed stomach was sagging a bit; started doing 100 leg lifts at Red Rocks	April 2012	ongoing	Definition in stomach returned and improved

I close this chapter on accomplishments with my best illustration of progress. I've shown this picture to many people. It always receives responses of amazement to what I was able to accomplish over a period of six months.

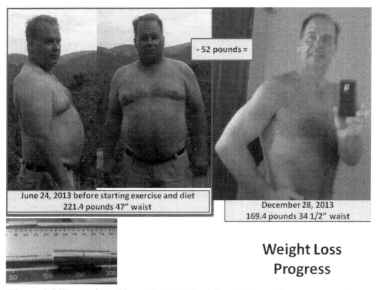

Figure 9 I Wanted to Close Out 2013 with a Picture. I went on to Lose 7 More Pounds and Bulk Up More

3. MOTIVATION

Guys tend to look at a woman's physique which prompts the woman to say, "My eyes are up here." A desirable physique could have men reversing the trend to where they would have to say this to a woman who is mesmerized by their body.

Motivation is the most difficult lifestyle change to implement as well as being the most difficult area to write about. Motivating yourself is covered in detail and maybe even too much detail. I do tend to over emphasize in this chapter however realize that it takes a lot of little things to add up to a successful effort in motivating yourself. I present many different ways to remain motivated in hopes you can implement the ones that work for you.

As I mentioned in the Foreword, this book has a dark side where I am egotistical and vain. You will see this emerge in the my illustration of what motivated me. This self-centered attitude cost me one relationship and was affecting my current relationship. As I wrote this book and became more aware of what my journey was really teaching me, I realized that my end success was more based on mental happiness than physical achievement. A different man emerged and to tell you the truth,

I didn't like the vain man that I portray here. As a result, I almost canned the whole project. I only saved this effort because I realized that I could share a success story on how I achieved happiness, and fitness rather than my initial goal of becoming a babe magnet that sought attention from all women. Believe me, the attention of one woman is enough if you are lucky enough to find the right woman like I did. Of course I still like the attention that a fit body gives me however my true happiness comes from the time spent with a person who appreciates the whole me, not just the physical me. She has taught me so much about inner as well as outer beauty. I now work to improve both. The physical success was the bridge to this overall improvement. Realize that as vain as I sound in the beginning of this chapter the journey ultimately leads to improved happiness. I thought good looks would bring me happiness. In the end, it led me to internal pride and happiness and a relationship that provided more happiness than I ever imagined. Still, the vain person that I was while achieving this goal had a lot to do with my success. No matter how much I wanted to cut that person out of the story, he was a true motivator during certain parts of my success. I hope you don't suffer too much with my ego here before you get to the parts where I understand the true value of this journey.

Because the success of your journey is mostly due to mental rather than physical efforts, there has to be a lot of emphasis on keeping you focused mentally by presenting ways to remain motivated. Presenting them is one thing. Providing logical flow for something as fragmented as motivation proved a bit more difficult. I found that the motivating factors I experienced were so intertwined and complicated that it was difficult to write this chapter with logical flow. No matter how many times I edited this chapter, it still appeared to be a jumbled mess. There are however some key points to be learned. Focus more on the lessons than the flow and you will get the gist of this chapter.

In this chapter I present a number of factors and then relate them to motivation. I am employing a method used by successful people; look for the opportunity and then act on it if you wish to achieve your goals. The opportunity to motivate yourself lies within the many facets associated with your lifestyle change. I evaluated these factors and realized each facet could be associated with a method within my lifestyle change and related to how I motivated myself. I take little pieces and add them up so that you will be able to overcome the unnatural desire to motivate yourself.

This chapter does have redundancies as a I relate topics to motivation. I do this on purpose. Motivation is not as simple as saying "I'm going to do this." Although that thought should be your underlying cause, motivation is a complicated subject that is initiated in many ways rather than by one single mode of operation.

We all have a certain form of physical ability. We also waste a lot of that physical ability by not motivating ourselves mentally to be active and eat healthy rather than to satisfy hunger and taste buds. We tend to revert to easier tasks and that induces laziness. Motivation pushes us beyond laziness. Triggering and maintaining motivation takes effort in itself. Effort is often opposite the human's desire to be lazy. We will resort to this more satisfying lazy lifestyle naturally. So how does one motivate a person when it is unnatural? The answer lies in understanding how we relate to motivation.

Humans are very complicated from a mental standpoint. We have a lot of thinking capability. Our minds and bodies seek pleasure in many different ways from many different inputs. Combine this complication with the many situations and distractions we encounter and it's apparent that it is difficult to focus on any one thing let alone focusing on a subject like motivation that requires effort as well. In addition to being complicated, we become bored easily. When this happens, we look for new ways to achieve pleasure. In summary, the complications and ever changing direction of the human mind is the basis that helps us to identify the opportunity to motivate ourselves in the various areas or facets of our lives.

Like the human's complicated mental thought processes, motivation is very complicated too. There is no single method for motivating people. I discovered this during my fitness journey. Motivation comes in small pieces that we have to assemble into the drive that moves us in the correct direction as we take this fitness journey.

Even if we do find a method to motivate, we can become bored with it. Therefore something that motivates us now might not motivate us in the future. This makes motivation rely on continuously changing the methods you pursue to remain motived. That is why I present so many little subjects to motivate you. These subjects occurred at different times during my journey. As I became bored with one method, I'd focus on other methods to remain motivated. Although it may seem like I'm throwing you at them all at once, what I am really doing is summarizing the opportunities I discovered to motivate myself and keep going. Picture it as a car that you want to drive 500,000 miles. The tires, belts, brakes, and other associated parts are going to wear out at different times. They won't all fail at the same time. Motivation is the same way. Opportunities to motivate yourself will appear at different times like they did for me. As you get bored, opportunities will disappear and you will have to discover new ways to remain motivated. I am presenting the story on how I found opportunities in my lifestyle methods for remaining motivated in order to achieve success.

Motivating yourself to get started on activities or eating healthy is a key task to making progress. As humans, we like to procrastinate and put off unpleasant tasks. Instead of starting off with how to motivate yourself, I present the results and work backwards.

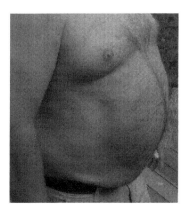

Figure 10 Before I Had a Large Overhang

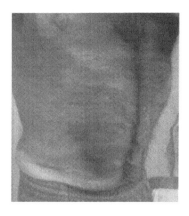

Figure 11 My Main Motivation was a Muscular, Flat, Stomach

The real motivation for losing weight is the success that you achieve. Often times this appears to be easy to say yet hard to do. Staying motivated is really more or less about being persistent and patient in the long run while being happy throughout the process.

My lifestyle methods that presented opportunities to remain motivated include

- Being aware of your progress
- How motivation fuels itself
- The roll of a lifestyle change in regards to motivation
- Staying motivated without enhancements or supplements
- Having a positive workout environment
- Not overdoing it
- Counting reps
- Celebrating your success
- Eating Habits
- Using dating and socialization to motivate
- Scheduling your activities in a manner that motivates
- The role of partners in motivating yourself
- Dealing with fatigue factors and plateaus

Maintaining awareness of your progress helps to motivate you. The biggest motivating factor is for you and others to physically see that you've improved. You won't stick with it if you don't see results. Therefore, it is important to keep track of your progress. Keeping track can be comprised of many things including recording your weight and dimensions. I wished I had kept closer track of my progress than I did. I weighed myself almost daily however I was told that it can result in disappointment so I didn't record the weight as frequently. I often experienced disappointment when I saw no results after working hard. By waiting longer periods to record results, more weight was lost due to time. This motivated me because you tend to go up and down on a daily basis due to a number of things including water intake. By not recording on a daily basis, I wasn't reminded of where I was yesterday especially if I had gone up in weight. I had a steady downward progression in weight loss that was more apparent when weighing myself over a longer period than daily. This method worked for me. Find a method of weighing yourself that keeps you motivated.

They say to weigh yourself at the same time every day. I would weigh myself upon rising in the morning. I would wait until after I went to the bathroom and weigh myself before I drank or ate. This method worked best for me. In previous weight loss efforts I would weigh myself before and after my lunch time workout. I would typically lose three pounds during the workout which was mostly water weight. I only weighed myself in the morning this time around. I didn't gauge workout activity as I believed a daily measure was a better indicator than the up and down nature of book ending my workout with weigh ins. Water adds weight. I didn't regulate my water intake every day so naturally I'd put on more water weight on the days I drank more. I focused more on quenching my thirst than on my amount of water consumption. As it turned out, the water helped me lose weight while spreading out the recording of my weight helped keep my motivation at a higher level.

In addition to weighing myself at a certain time relative to certain activities, I also made sure I wore the same amount of clothing every time I weighted. For me, I always record my weight while wearing just a pair of shorts such as briefs or swimming trunks. This way I was void of additional weight due to the clothing, shoes, belts, and anything in the pockets such as cell phones.

In the same way that weighing myself proved to be a motivator, measuring myself did too. I spread the measurements of my body out over longer periods as I knew progress would take weeks if not months. This method of measuring my dimensions over a longer period was also a key motivator. I also lost size as muscle gave way to fat. I tend to use visual motivation for certain areas versus measuring size. I wasn't as religious about measuring my progress in areas such as my waist, chest, and arms. Instead I monitored progress in the mirror. I knew the routine I was performing was likely to reduce my size in these areas especially when I was in the weight loss phase where I was lifting lighter weight at higher repetitions and lower weight. What amazed me however was that I lost over an inch around my cheeks. I lost so much weight in my neck that I had wrinkles become more pronounced under my chin. I grew a beard to hide these wrinkles. Overall, my face looked thinner and did develop some lines. I'll take the more mature, thinner look over the fat baby face any day.

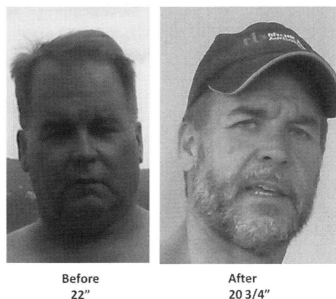

Before	After
22"	20 3/4"

Figure 12 My Face Diameter Shrunk 1 ¼ Inches

Weighing yourself is a good way to judge progress however the best scale is the mirror. Seeing results first hand is the best way to motivate yourself next to compliments from those who see and notice your improvements. Because compliments come randomly and unexpectedly, the mirror is the best regular indication of your progress as it provides a daily monitoring and comparison method. It's invigorating to see the toning of the body as muscle definition appears where smooth fat once existed. The mirror provides you with this opportunity.

Watching a toned body emerge is a huge motivator. Going from fat to fit is visually rewarding and satisfying. It's an amazing thing to realize that is really your body and not someone else's that you are viewing in the mirror.

When I see a pendulous belly now, I think, "That's easy to fix."

A year ago, it seemed like such an insurmountable achievement. I never thought I would have a flat stomach. Motivation and lifestyle change allowed me to reach a level of abdominal muscle definition I never thought possible. If I can do it, anybody can, especially you the reader.

For me the best visual improvement was the V shape of my torso emerging. I had accomplished body transitions before however I never really lost my stomach and love handles. This time around, I was able to expand my back muscles and shrink my waist to a point where I developed a nice V shape with my lats sloping inwards down towards by waist. It helped that I also increased my lat size as well as reducing my waist and love handles. This provided a wider upper torso at chest level which combined nicely with the smaller diameter of my waist resulting in a V shaped body that tapered from my shoulders to my hips.

My stomach went from a paunchy beer gut with love handles to a concaved indent below my ribs with an island of muscle along the center. Although I longed for a six pack, I refused to shave my chest and stomach in order to see if it emerged. I'm not that fanatical about my body. Still, I was able to view the occasional shadow that showed muscular ripple indicating a six pack might be there after all. I eliminated my protruding, rounded abdomen and replaced it with one that is flat and muscular. The overhang is gone and it feels great. I have more range of motion with something as simple as tying my shoes. Before, if something fell on the floor when I was seated on a plane, I'd have to wait until we landed and stood up in order to retrieve it. Now it's just a matter of bending forward in the seat. I'm also able to get into more positions when retrieving items from cabinets or during sex. Did he just say that? Yeah I did. I'm presenting results on how fitness makes you more appealing. Improving your ability to perform sexual activity is one of the main motivators. If you don't believe me, ask your partner.

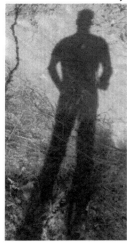

Figure 13 Mr. Vain and His "V" Shape

I work out in a mirror if I can. This offers both benefits and some disappointment as well. Remember, progress comes slow and it will sometimes appear as if you aren't progressing when you actually are. A mirror helps show your body emerging. Different light and movements will profile your muscular structure. As you work out, you will begin to notice progress as muscle builds and definition takes place. I transitioned from stringy "old man" muscles and moobs (man boobs) that pointed to the floor to a defined and toned body with perky pectorals. My pectorals are round and protruding as a result of the various angles of presses that I perform on the incline bench. My shoulders now slope nicely from my neck. They are rounded with definition where once they were smooth and somewhat saggy. My stomach is defined and has ripples. My ribs are showing. I have definitions in my arms in the front (biceps) as well as the back (triceps). There are "cuts" in my shoulders; indentations that show the muscular definition. All of this appeared in larger proportions than I would have thought possible at age 52. I once heard that a man starts losing muscle at age forty yet here I exist more defined and bigger than I was in my 20's and 30's. Protein and activity worked for me! I'm proof that it's never too late in life to get fit and add tone. The ability to grow muscle size and transition a saggy body that once looked old motivates me.

The mirror helped me in other ways. Believing my abdominal work was no longer effective, I had slacked off a bit. When I looked in the mirror I noticed my stomach was sagging. I immediately increased my reps and days for abdominals. Within days, the sagging had receded. I still didn't have a sideways "V" shape from my back to my waist. I began some back exercises that enlarged my inner back muscles and soon developed the "V". To my amazement, I could feel the small of my back was no longer touching the bench. This improvement occurred within the first few sets of doing back exercises. It motivated me to know results can be achieved this quickly.

In addition to visual monitoring, compliments are a huge motivator. They bring awareness to your progress.

It makes the effort so well worth it to experience these compliments. The positive nature of the feedback is a huge motivator. Negativity turns us off. By seeking compliments, the positive feedback motivated me. I went a little overboard on this quest and became vain. In the end however, it was a key part of my journey in terms of motivating me to achieve.

The most memorable improvement of all was the reaction from women. Lately I can't go a week without a woman commenting on my body. These compliments come from those who knew me in my past when I was heavy as well as from those who have met me for the first time. If someone who never met you notices your physique and compliments you, it is a huge motivator as they have no former reference point from which to gauge your progress. It's as if your success is even more obvious. I can't tell you how many times I've turned heads due to having trimmed my body. This never happened when I was out of shape and overweight. One lady that was seated on a bench in downtown Scottsdale even started clapping as I approached shirtless while tanning on a winter trip. I never said a word to her. Instead, I smiled and bounced my right pectoral muscle a few times. The next day, two women stopped me on Squaw Peak, a trail in Phoenix, Arizona. They both complimented my body. They were surprised to learn I was 52 years old. Now that I'm adding muscle, I'm getting a lot of compliments on my arms. This motivates me even further. You too will notice that compliments incentivize you to keep going and even pursue progress with more vigor.

I've even had men compliment me on my size and definition. It makes me want to go work out even more as men are typically not complimentary of other men. Compliments are the best motivators. Seek them, enjoy them, keep generating them. Compliments and attention are desired human interactions. Think about it this way, birthdays make us happy. This is an example of humans liking attention. Motivation comes from things you like of which attention is a likable interaction. Use it to your advantage.

I'm sharing these welcome occurrences with readers in order to inspire you to enjoy the success I have. Being fit really does bring out compliments and portray you as younger than your years. Compliments will motivate you so invite them into your life without feeling like you are being vain. Some may view presenting or discussing your progress and size increase as being vain however are you really doing this so that you will go unnoticed? Of course not. Enjoy the compliments you receive and subtly seek them as rewards that motivate you to improve even further. Compliments supplement and increase happiness. Happiness brings even more interest in you. In my case it has resulted in me obtaining some new friends. They were drawn in by my happy nature. Now I have more potential workout buddies that were enticed by my happiness and physique while being motivated by the success I have had.

All of these episodes were gratifying and welcoming rewards for a hard earned respect. I never garnered so much as a look when I was overweight and pudgy. Now people were going out of their way to mention the definition of my muscles. The motivating factor was that the progress was obvious to people other than myself. I was achieving success for the hard work and it was getting noticed. Regardless of how egotistical it may appear, few people work hard without seeking results. Results drive us to produce more and better results. I have found this to be true on my journey. The more people compliment, the harder I work. Employ this same method to motivate yourself to improve. People will see the new you and mention the difference. What are you waiting for? Start now, not next week.

I purposely wore tight shirts in order to best showcase my body. You will also feel better as your body challenges the material by stretching it to a point where the definition pushes through the fabric. Although this appears to be egotistical or self absorbed, realize that you worked damn hard for that body, so why would you hide it under bulky clothes? Do people cover up tattoos? No, they display them. By displaying your body with fitted clothing, the reaction from others will help motivate you to maintain and improve. When you hide your body, you are removing potentially motivating comments.

I would much rather sport a chiseled body than have to invade my body with needles that produce a tattoo in order for people to identify with me or find my body interesting. I look at it this way: showcasing a muscular body is my way of displaying art in a manner similar to others who choose tattoos to do so. We are both doing the same thing as well as seeking attention. So why view displaying a hard body as being vain? It's no different than displaying a tattoo, piercings, or jewelry or wearing a shirt with a saying on it. Besides, don't you men want to say "my eyes are up here" like women say to you? This could happen if a babe found your body enticing enough to gaze upon it. It never happened when I was chubby. It happens now that I have a muscular chest protruding above a flat stomach.

Transitioning your workout routine will provide motivation especially as you reach plateaus. The first six months of my work I focused on losing weight by doing high repetitions with lower weight. I lost a lot of size in my arms, chest, and waist as the fat melted away. However I hit a plateau on weight loss. I decided to start putting bulk on in the form of muscle.

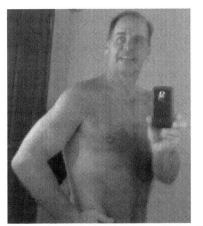 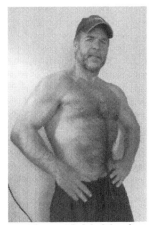

Figure 14 I Was Lanky When Using 25 lb Dumb Bells

Figure 15 My Muscle Definition Improved With the 45 lb Dumb Bells

As my journey transitioned from a weight loss effort to an effort to achieve more muscle definition, I took a different approach than when I was younger. Back then it was always about improving strength and the amount of weight I could push. Now I wanted to remain fit without over taxing my body.

I decided to start with light weights and low repetitions. By doing so, I burned fat quickly while slowly getting my body used to the weights as they stressed previously unused muscles, ligaments, and tendons. This did two things. First it conditioned my body at a rate that avoided injury. Second it allowed me to enjoy the workouts as they were doable. I wasn't stressed about moving up in weight. I had a feeling of accomplishment by achieving my desired 50 and 100 repetitions.

Nothing will set you back quicker than an injury. As you age, you will heal at a slower pace. Therefore, it is important to acclimate your body to the additional stress slowly by using this method of light weight and high repetitions. Transition to higher repetitions and weight after properly preparing your body. Never push through an exercise by using improper form or throwing the weights. If you can't perform the activity with a slow steady movement, break into more sets or lower the weight. Finally, settle on higher weight with lower repetitions if you want muscular size.

My workouts with lighter weight and more repetitions proved

enjoyable. I wasn't seeing how many reps I could do at a certain weight. For example, I didn't increase the weight and lower the reps. I focused on getting 50 or 100 reps comfortably at a doable amount of weight. Attempting to move the amount of weight up constantly had yielded a series of highs and lows in my past. Along with it came demotivating disappointment. Instead I knew my goals and was able to achieve them with a minimal amount of pain and discomfort. There is always some of discomfort however I kept it to the level of a "good hurt" where the pain was actually motivational to a point that it felt good. I didn't push myself to a level of discomfort and disappointment. My body actually wanted it more in most cases. This was most prevalent in my abdomen where couldn't seem to do enough. I had never experienced this before. In the past, this area had always seemed to be difficult and painful to work to a point where I gave up. My body taught me that there is a hump to get over. On the other side lies a desirable situation where the muscle actually craves more activity. This pleasant discovery motivated me. Your body has the same capability. My advice is to pursue it to a point where you find it. I'm a regular person just like you are. If I can achieve this level, anybody can.

Remember, motivation and success each require patience. Bring your body up to speed at a pace that it can handle. Tendons, ligaments, bone, and muscles strengthen with use. Lower weight stresses them less. Start with lighter weight and increase as you "outgrow" their effectiveness and your body strengthens to a point where it can handle the additional weight.

After about six months of activity, I was thin and lanky. I had achieved goals I never thought possible in terms of weight loss and now it was time to set new ones. This was vital to motivating myself to improve further. Now I had achieved success on this incredible journey, I sought to add to it. I wanted to increase the size as well as definition of my muscles. I moved to heavier dumb bells as a method for growing muscle size and definition. I progressed from 15 pounders, to 20 pounders, and then finally to 45 pounders in most areas. I remained with 20 pounders in areas that I felt were taxing my body too much because I was after a physique and not strength. I'm 52 years old, my strong years are behind me. I have implemented a routine that my body can handle. Had I done that in earlier years, I would not have created the back injury that slightly paralyzes my leg.

Note that in my younger years I used dumb bells of up to 70 pounds with wrist straps to help suspend the weights. I am achieving better definition with the lighter, 45 pounders while the stress on my joints is far less. This is a key transition for my older body as my number one source of pain is tendon and ligament stress. I listen to my body and appease it. I avoid the painful in favor of the activities that produce pain free benefits some of which caused me to desire additional activity. In this manner, I stay motivated. Your lifestyle change will be easier to implement if you follow this method of making workouts enjoyable.

As I researched the competition for this book I noticed several things. Those touting weight loss and fitness over 50 were body builders, triathletes, and gym rats. Furthermore, their clients tended to be of the same nature. There appeared to be no gray area in fitness. They all had chiseled bodies with little or no fat. There was really no material for a regular guy seeking fitness without an atlas body. The majority of the information was for competitive bodybuilding.

After the success I achieved I came to the same conclusion that I had for all of my weight loss efforts. There has to be a balance in life between fitness and happiness. I failed to achieve this balance in the past which is part of the reason I regained the weight. I had starved my way to success yet I couldn't maintain that lifestyle. For me, a low carb, protein based menu kept me satisfied and fulfilled.. The result with this latest effort is that I have both fitness and happiness. For me the desire was to have larger and more defined looks while enjoying life rather than to have the ultimate body that my competition preaches. My end desire is what sets this book apart from the competition. I'm not pushing you to a body that is worthy of competitive showcasing with the likelihood you will become overwhelmed and quit. I'm introducing a lifestyle with balance that will more likely keep you motivated. I am also providing you with natural ways to transition your lifestyle without pushing gimmicks and supplements that are profit based. Instead, this was an economical if not profitable venture for me. I hope you realize the same success.

Competitive body builders look freaky to me. I actually think stringy muscle is gross to look at. Therefore, I like to maintain a certain amount of fat in order to smooth over the stringy look. I actually feel that stringy muscles, veins, and tendons poking through your skin also looks unhealthy. We were meant to have a certain percentage of body fat. In some instances this can be attractive. For me, babies with body fat are more attractive than skinny babies. Also I discovered that losing fat to a certain point is easy. The closer you get to the stringy look, the harder it gets.

Achieving a competitive body takes a lot of effort; more effort than most of us have time for. Achievement of this level requires dedication that results in a loss of balance in life. Although there is a certain level of dedication required to achieve my results, I tried to have a happy life without being obsessed to the point of being fanatical. I don't want to compete, I just want to feel good about myself and presentation in addition to being healthy. Thus I have written this book not as a sculpted gym rat with a perfect body as much as from the standpoint of the regular guy who wants to be healthy and attractive while enjoying life. If you want a drill sergeant to beat you into competitive form, there are plenty out there. I am not one of them. This book is more about achieving attainable goals and happiness than having the perfect body. By taking a journey similar to mine, you will still get the compliments and feel better yet the task won't be so overwhelming that you lose motivation. It is ok to strive for a body worthy of competing in bodybuilding contest however for the most part, it's unobtainable unless you are extremely dedicated and for the most part, obsessed. If the lifestyle change consumes you too much, you will tend to ignore other aspects of your life and therefore will not maintain the lifestyle as frustration will set in as balance is lost requiring to sacrifice more and more. My methods are about taking a happy journey, not imposing an intimidating sentence. As with anything, there has to be balance. That is what this book is about; having a balance in achieving fitness while enjoying life.

Weighing myself was essential to gauging progress during my loss phase as well as when I was adding muscle. What was amazing was that I continued to lose weight even when I was lifting the heavier dumbbells in my effort to bulk up. The increased size and definition combined with the continued weight loss further motivated me. Although I measured a final loss of 59 pounds, I believe my actual body transition was somewhere around 70 to 75 pounds when you consider the amount of muscle that I gained. Muscle is more dense than fat so it stands to reason that I took off weight with fat loss yet put on a higher ratio of weight with muscle gain. Therefore my overall weight transition was beyond my total weight loss in pounds. I saw motivation continuously boosting itself when I bulked up while losing weight. I have addressed the way motivation fuels itself continuously in this paragraph. My journey reveled the fact that motivation does not always come from within someone who is continuously pushing themselves. Rather it is like a turbo booster on a car where the more exhaust pressure you generate the more air you spool into the engine further improving its performance. Motivation can be like a spark that ignites a fire that fuels itself. Achieving this level of motivation will make your journey much easier than you think. It is within you. Find it like I did and become happier like I am.

Find motivation in how your body responds to your lifestyle change. The key element in my transition was an overall lifestyle change that involved activity and nutrition. My routine and eating habits were adding muscle while continuing to burn fat. I was progressing in my desired direction which motivated me further. The fat that remained or was ingested was still being turned into energy. I was taking in very few carbs so my body turned to itself as a source of energy. The protein in my food was turning into muscle due to the workouts. I had found the combination for success that had so often eluded me in my previous weight loss efforts when I failed to scale back my carb intake and on alcohol. I was having fun and enjoying my routine, while still feeling full and satisfied as well as energetic. This was very motivational.

When a commenter on Facebook accused me of taking steroids, I proudly responded, "That's all effort and protein, son. I've never done an illegal drug in my life."

That's partially true now that I think about it. I have never ingested or injected an illegally drug in my life. I did cave to peer pressure and also wanted to impress a girl so I tried marijuana. I did not like the way it made me feel like I lost control of my mental abilities so twice was enough for a lifetime. Besides, lungs don't like smoke so why put smoke in them? You wouldn't stay in a burning building if you couldn't breathe due to smoke, would you? Get a clue. Your body is telling you something. Stop smoking; everything. You will become fit faster if you have full use of your lungs. Don't impede them with anything. Don't use enhancements either.

My achievements were obtained without using any form of enhancement. I have my own opinion about enhancements. Suffice it to say I believe they are unnecessary. I'm not about to ingest or inject foreign substances for gain especially when I have achieved success by focusing on protein based nutrition that my body implemented by rebuilding muscle that I tore down with the weights. I'd rather work a little harder than cut any corners in order to accelerate gains. To me, it's a personal choice based on the individual. However, I'm not about to make gains now and pay for it later in life. Altering the body has serious consequences as many body builders have discovered. I never did supplements or drugs. I'm happy I didn't as I took on this effort at a time in life where many people my age are dragging around oxygen bottles. It was motivating for me to know that I could achieve results through activity and food choices without having to take enhancements or follow fads. I proved that fitness is entirely possible while maintaining your health and avoiding supplements. I doubt you are that different from me where you cannot achieve the same results. Don't take short cuts. Ask the Donner party.

I didn't become so focused on my food intake that it became unpleasant to a point where I was no longer motivated. I used some basic rules of limiting my food class to low carbs and then tried different combinations to see what worked and what didn't. Experiment to find your success point. Don't get hooked into a stringent routine that worked for one person. This is a journey. Take different roads to see what works and more importantly, what motivates progress. Note that I experimented with various combinations of activites and foods. The activities were for developing a certain part of my body and enhancing my stamina. The foods were nutrition that I needed yet they offered a method for losing weight and adding muscle. I didn't follow a stringent set of recipes, menu, quantities, and regulation like so many other weight loss books tell you to do. I ate until I was satisfied yet I ate "smart" in terms of the content of my food. Although those routines may have worked for the authors, a stringent regiment is seldom the right combination for everyone. You get to the right combination for a fit body by implementing the methods described in this book instead of following a restricted regiment that worked for a certain individual. The results require a bit of trial and error. Be patient. It will help you avoid frustration which could result in a loss or reduction of motivation.

In the beginning I started recording my intake. I quickly became bored with that. I realized that this was not a mathematical effort rather it was a lifestyle change where I had to have an overall awareness versus micro monitoring everything I ate and programming my meals to the extent of being anal about it. Instead of regimenting each meal, I focused on my overall carb intake as well as the carb content of the foods I kept around. By simplifying my approach, I eased my stress which motivated me further. I felt less restricted as the time consuming aspect of detailed monitoring was now absent. If I was going to be anal about anything, it was going to be maintaining and improving on my activity level. My time was better spent burning calories by being active than by fretting about my numbers. This method of burning fat versus worrying about how much I ingested worked for me. Finding the right combination will work for you. Be patient and monitor your progress for results at a pleasing interval. If it isn't working after about three weeks, then change it up. Worrying about it on a daily basis for me was too taxing mentally. It isn't delightful and is demotivating. I tossed the tendency to over analyze my intake and was more successful.

Your activity environment is very crucial to maintaining motivation. Having a pleasing environment is motivational. Introducing variety while looking for new opportunities will keep your routines fresh and desirable.

Although I have consistent workout places and routines, I'm not limited to them. I constantly look for opportunities to do both aerobic activity and muscle building! I expanded my routine at Red Rocks as I observed others. I added upper body activities to the leg workouts the stair climbing offered. I've even used my luggage and the furniture in an airport as a mini gymnasium. I took advantage of early arrival time at the airport. Instead of sitting on my duff I found areas without people present and snuck in a few dips, curls, sit ups, and arm extensions.

I wish to reemphasize my desire to be outdoors as one of the environmental factors that I use to motivate myself. I am less motivated when confined to inside activities. I seek outdoor activity and tolerate indoor activity. I often move my weights and equipment outside to work out on the deck when weather permits. I've had to move snow off my equipment and the deck when I want to work out. Nothing stands in my way. By limiting the excuses, I increase my chances at success. The success and feeling of accomplishment despite the odds motivational.

Optimizing your routine for pleasant outdoor experiences will motivate you to do more activities. I watch the weather and know the days I can work out outside or inside and then plan accordingly. I even watch the weather on a time of day basis so that I can catch the more favorable times. For example, if it's going to be sunny in the morning and cloudy in the afternoon I will adjust my schedule so that my outdoor portion occurs during the most favorable weather. I keep extra workout clothes in my car so that I can take advantage of an opportunity to perform an aerobic activity. I even climb stairs in dress pants and shoes. I eliminate excuses to avoid activity as they will keep me from being motivated and achieving my goals.

It is essential to make your routine as well as your environment enjoyable and something that'll you'll look forward to such as the scenery of my deck where I lifted weights. For me, my aerobics portion was enjoyable due beauty of the overlook I hiked to on Bergen Mountain and the stunning backdrop of Red Rocks amphitheater where I climbed stairs. Aesthetic beauty is a motivator. Rocky motivated himself even without this. In the movie, he awoke and ran through the dismal, gray city. This is one of the most motivational movie scenes ever created. What helped the scene the most? The music that was played in the background. It's hard to listen to the Rocky theme without feeling motivated. Find music that works in the same manner and listen to it during your activities in order to motivate yourself.

It's not always possible to perform your activity portion in a scenic location. If you don't have access to an amphitheater or slope to climb, a stadium or high school bleachers serve the same purpose. Indoor stair cases work well during periods of bad weather. They also can fill the void when on travel.

I have two forms of stair climbs; individual stairs and "two at a time". This tends to achieve the best results for me. The lifting action of doing more stairs per single step has made me much stronger and improved my stamina. The ability to climb using either method without stopping is a motivating factor for me. I feel like I've accomplished something because I'm no longer stopping to rest.

It helped that Red Rocks is a mecca for exercise especially among ladies. We tend to be more motivated by the presence of the opposite sex. Being surrounded by activity really boosts the spirits and desire to succeed. When the majority of people around you are working out, you get incentivized. The variety of activity going on at Red Rocks also provided a few clues on different methods of exercises that has helped me further improve specific areas of my body. Gymnasiums offer a similar mix of activity and the opposite sex. If that environment motivates you then by all means use it. It was once a motivator for me as well.

Even more fun was realized when I scheduled to meet my dates at Red Rocks for a workout. It provided an additional motivating factor as I got to see the person as well as complete my routine. Accomplishing two tasks at once is in itself motivational. Having venues that are appealing and invigorating will motive you as well. My dates have now progressed to hiking as a form of motivational activities. I have seen some of the most beautiful places in the Rocky Mountains. Experiencing these areas with someone that you care about is even better. I'm motivated by the scenery and the companionship.

A key motivational suggestion is to not overdo it. I took entire days off! Nobody is capable of working out every day. By averaging my activity over certain days, I kept losing weight. The same success is occurring during my maintenance phase. I've found that I can hit my major three muscle areas; back, chest, and shoulders; once a week while still maintaining my level of fitness. From there, I back fill the muscle development and maintenance with aerobic activities. Because these are regularly scheduled parts of my lifestyle, I remain motivated to keep on course rather than skipping them and being lazy. I have achieved a balance that keeps me happy and fit. I neither overdo it or under do it.

Scheduling is important to maintaining motivation in other ways. Life's events and even the weather can affect when you perform your activities. Look both ahead and behind at your schedule. If I haven't done certain activities in the last few days, they go to the top priority on my list. For me these areas are weight lifting for increasing muscle size and definition and aerobic activity for burning weight as well as improving stamina. I intermingle these areas with abdominal activities. I often combine a muscle development day with abdominal exercises. I'll combine an aerobics day with abdominal exercises as well. On some days I've done all three areas when I've had time. My success has settled on isolating the aerobic and weight days while making abdominals more regularly scheduled. I think a lot of this has to do with my desire to always have a muscular abdomen. I also have wanted to avoid having a belly now that I've achieved my lifetime dream of being near six pack abs. I give the biggest muscles in my body the most attention. At Red Rocks I combine stair climbing with upper body and abdominal workouts. This combines muscle development and aerobic activities. The repetitions that I do for my abdominals as well as my muscle development each elevate my breathing and aerobic, calorie burning activity. The aerobic activity expands my lungs so that I can do more reps. All of these factors are intertwined to a point where they benefit each other. Motivation is a key part of it.

There will be times when you just have to push yourself even if you have properly scheduled your work outs. Don't let your workout be the last thing on your list. Schedule it along with the other tasks that you have to complete and be sure to make it a priority rather than optional. If it's optional, you'll be less likely to complete it and more likely to skip it. This only hurts you as progress requires execution to the point of completion. Strive for perfection and you will achieve excellence (as per motivational coach, Vince Lombardi). And it is so worth the effort. Keep going and the results will come. Give up and you will become soft and regain the weight. Motivate yourself by remaining determined and keeping your appointments with yourself. Don't let the despair of missing your workout demotivate your efforts. Have the balance where you miss other things that are less important.

Scheduling has other aspects of importance. Some activities such as eating, showering, and dressing are daily tasks that can't be pushed aside. Other tasks are based on completion dates such as annual taxes. Realize that you can only do so much in a day. Make sure that you don't schedule too many activities and that your workout is a part of it. Trying to do too much results in missed deadlines and disappointment. Under estimate and over achieve. Don't overwhelm yourself. Have a schedule that is relaxed rather than making you uptight and edgy. After all, you are only human. Trying to be super human will result in failure. Being realistic will result in achieving and surpassing goals. The success that results will motivate you. Defeat and failure will not.

If you have to cut corners, find less beneficial areas and cut those out of your schedule while still being able to complete your activity. For me, I sacrificed meal time, TV, and social time and kept time for activity. Instead of taking time to prepare and sit down to a formal meal, I ate premade meals while at my computer or while just standing in the kitchen. If I cooked, I used the oven heat to make several meals that I sometimes heated up quickly in the microwave over the span of a week. I spent less time eating and more time performing an activity (remember, we don't like the words diet and exercise). The important part to me was the exercise so it received the priority over relaxed dining. The same went for TV. I would even exercise while in bed or on the phone. Put your phone on speaker or use ear buds. Mute the mic in order to mask your breathing that will elevate as a result of the activity. No matter what the situation, I kept moving and kept improving. It paid off big time. Hell yeah it took energy and initiation yet I ended up being more energetic and motivated to a point where it required less initiative on my part. Steal time for your workout and enjoy the success that motivates instead of cheating yourself which results in demotivating guilt and shame.

Partners help motivate you too. If you have a partner with integrity, they will be less inclined to cancel on you at the last minute. You've asked for that person's time and now you have a certain sense of obligation as well. Use this as a motivator. Believe it or not, one of my motivating friends is a person on Facebook I've never met in person. She lives in another state. She posts her workout accomplishments and I compliment her on progress. She also compliments on mine. Facebook has resulted in me motivating a few other friends too who in turn motivate me. Posting the occasional picture of my progress also solicits motivational compliments. To my Facebook family I'm a regular guy with a regular life they have been a part of in some way in a past life. I'm not some super human celebrity. When my friends see my accomplishments, they tend to believe they can do the same. We tend to pull each other along. Social media in general is a motivator. I've recently expanded to a website, blog, youtube, twitter, and I'm writing article for LinkedIn and a fitness website shapefit.com. I have to have to constantly generate new things to tell my audience which motivates me to keep active and on my successful food intake.

Numbers and counting repetitions play a huge part in motivation especially when you consider I was doing on the order of 50 and 100 reps per exercise. It may sound like a lot however you'd be surprised at how little time they take. You can knock out 500 reps during the 20 minutes of commercials in an hour long TV show. The best way to approach a quantity of this magnitude (50 to 100) is to break down the repetitions into smaller increments. I would do 50 then 30 then 20 to get to 100 reps. Similarly, I would do 30 and then 20 to get to 50 reps when I did heavier weights. By doing the larger amount first, you catch the muscle before it gets fatigued. Also, you get the bigger portion out of the way early which in itself is a motivator. Who eagerly accepts doing more work? Not most people. A lower number in the second set can become a motivating incentive to push onward toward completion.

Play games with your workout. Instead of counting up, count down to the number of remaining repetitions. If doing 50, don't look at 25 as half way. Instead, get to 30 and realize you only have 20 left. Typically, knocking out an additional 20 is easy for me especially if I'm counting down. I adopted 20 as my number. I had a girl I liked named Joanie so instead of saying 20 I'd say Joanie. It really helped. 21, 22, 23, etc. became Joanie-one, Joanie-two, Joanie-three. In order to do 50 reps, I'd get to thirty (after Joanie nine) and then start counting at one to get the next twenty (Joanie) in. Joanie once told me that achieving as six pack would get me anything I wanted. I kept that goal in mind even after we split. It kept me motivated in my quest for a six pack. I also promised her I'd stop drinking. I adopted the promise for myself. Whether or not she was still around, I had made a promise. As a man of integrity, it was up to me to keep the promise regardless of her presence in my life.

Another way to motivate yourself is to focus on the muscle. Instead of completing your repetitions as a task to achieve a certain number, experience every repetition. Isolate the muscle with your brain and feel it working. Slow down and work through the entire motion emphasizing both directions of movement while concentrating on the muscle. Our brains have the amazing ability to do this. This works very well for my curls. When I focus on my bicep I use a more effective motion and feel the muscle expanding. Use positive and negative directions equally in order to get the full benefit from each repetition. Surprisingly, slowing down isn't any harder and can be easier if you mentally follow the motion. If you find you can't complete the set, lower the number of repetitions and break it out over several sets. If the weight seems too difficult, do 20 with the heavier weight and 30 with a slightly lighter one. Keep going until you can do all 50 with the heavier weight. Focus on progress and the results will come! Eventually you will come to a combination of repetitions, sets, and weight that will work for you. Expect plateaus yet realize you will gradually improve. If not, try something new until you do. Your body does have limits and you will hit plateaus. How you incorporate these limits will have a lot to do with staying motivated.

Sometimes I'll lose track of where I am when counting. As a method of achieving the next level, I always do more instead of less. If I do fewer, I'm only cheating myself. I have made great strides by pushing the envelope. There is no ceiling for me yet there is a floor. I never do under my minimum yet strive to do over my maximum.

The same goes with eating habits. I tend to revert to my successful food group while not cheating. If I do have the occasional sugary snack, I keep it in my mouth longer, get the pleasure from the taste, and then swallow after enjoying it. I don't eat sugary food in quantities as it becomes detrimental once it leaves your mouth. Women often say, "a minute on the lips is a lifetime on the hips". Prolong the pleasure in the area it is best experienced which is where the taste buds are in your mouth. You have nothing in your body after your mouth that experiences pleasure from sugar. Savor then swallow. That way you get the pleasure without the added calories like you do when you consume a sugary food for the purpose of satisfying hunger. If you must satisfy hunger, use fat or protein based foods. These tend to satisfy quicker in smaller quantities....at least for me that seems to be the situation.

Also note that calories is not a phrase I use very often in this book. I prefer to use carbs as in carbohydrates. Without getting into scientific terms, carbs are related to energy production and storage whereas calories are more related to a unit of measure for energy burned. Carbs and fat are energy sources. I focus on limiting the source versus figuring how to burn it off. This method has proved successful for me. Calories are tough to follow and monitor. They are burned off differently for each activity and their effect is not immediate. That's why it takes a few days to gain or lose weight based on your activity and intake. By averaging out your balance, you will see results. Trying to run five miles and then look for results only causes immediate gratification or disappointment. Weight loss is not an immediate result. Rather, it's averaged over time. So take time and be patient. Otherwise you will lose motivation.

There are other methods of motivation that I use. For instance I keep going through distractions. If an ear bud falls out, or a text arrives, or the music stops, I complete my reps prior to responding. I think of my buddy telling me about his days as a Marine. They were taught that slapping a bug could disclose the location of an entire regiment. Similarly, Vince Lombardi encouraged his men to live with the small hurts. Ignoring disturbances requires motivation yet it yields results. The same goes for irritants such as clothing or pinching skin when gripping a dumb bell. I gut through the discomfort and get to the other side. Unless I'm in danger of injuring myself, minor irritants are of minor importance so I dismiss them. Mental toughness results in achieving success quicker and at higher levels. This is a mental effort more than a physical. Use the mental to overcome the physical. Focus on completion rather than the distraction or discomfort. Motivate yourself to succeed.

I need to mention a phenomenon I call the fatigue factor. I believe our bodies produce chemicals which make us feel tired after a certain amount of activity. I noticed it at a particular place on the mountain when I hiked. My legs would start to ache at that location every time. Similarly, I would notice achiness at certain repetition numbers, usually around 20. I believe this was a fatigue point our bodies introduce that tell us to rest and preserve energy. Animals are very good at this. For instance, Cheetahs will break off a chase they judge as nonproducing in order to preserve energy. Humans do the same by saving energy for situations that may mean life or death. We are naturally inclined to rest rather than put forth effort. I believe this is a natural fatigue process for saving energy. It results in laziness being desirable over being active.

The key to motivating yourself is to work beyond the ache and feeling of fatigue. I found that the achy feeling will subside if it's due to activity and your body claiming fatigue. If it's due to injury, it's time to listen to your body and stop whatever is aggravating the injured area. Breaking through the pain takes your body to the next level of, "This flight/fight is for real." In other words, your body is being called upon to rescue itself from harm in some way rather than being pushed to unnecessarily burn precious energy. Adrenalin is the higher form in which the body gears up in response to danger. Because working out has no danger, no adrenalin is produce. You have to replace the adrenalin with by mentally incentivizing yourself through motivation. You do it every day for unpleasant tasks so why not do it for one that is fun, rewarding, and invigorating? The tired ache actually subsides after a certain amount of activity. Getting beyond this point is a motivation method that works very well. Expect the ache and keep going past it from fatigue to fight or flight. Program your mind to act as adrenalin that offsets the fatigue factor. Coaches do this with motivational speeches before taking the field, court, or rink. They build up the desire that fear normally creates as sort of an adrenelin.

Also mentally prepare your mind to know the achy fatigue feeling will eventually subside thus making the task more enjoyable. Succumbing to the ache and quitting is not an option if you are going to be successful. The phrase "hurts so good" actually applies to me. Some hurt feels good and I long to reproduce it. There is an area in my lower biceps that illicit this desire in me. Other hurts I ignore until they go away, which almost always happens. Then the endorphins kick in and I start to feel good. Everybody likes to feel good. Exercise will make you feel so much better. The desire to feel good in itself should motivate you. You just have to get over the fatigue hump if you want to get to the good feeling.

Don't quit whatever you do. The feeling of tiredness and achy muscles produce a desire to quit. If you quit you will never achieve your goals. Expect the pain and work through it and beyond it. Motivate yourself to overcome the desire to quit by wanting to succeed. As I tell my kids in regards to life, if it were easy, everybody would be doing it. Earn your right to be toned and desirable. Leave laziness to the overweight and undesirable. They will eventually cease to be competition as you sport a nice, hard body that turns heads and brings forth compliments. Nothing incentivizes you more than to feel a hard body as you soap yourself in the shower or having a lady hug you while feeling and complimenting your physique. For my female readers, us men notice that you don't jiggle when you wiggle. A toned body is highly desirable over flab. It really doesn't take much to lose weight once you find the right combination. You won't find it if you quit. You will however find it if you persist.

Expect to hit highs and lows in your workout. You will have that day where you feel tired and would rather skip your workout. Typically pushing yourself to be active will result in overcoming this feeling unless you have extremely exhausted your body. Admittedly, some days you need to listen to your body and rest. Most often however, you will feel better and be happy you were active despite feeling tired as the endorphins you produce provide a chemical feeling of satisfaction that tends to eliminate the tiredness. I'll admit that not being hung over also eliminates tiredness. I've been way more motivated since giving up alcohol entirely. I now get my buzz from endorphins more than the effects of alcohol.

Similarly, you will have a great day only to have it feel like you've lost progress the next time you workout. You won't be able to do as many reps or the weights will feel heavier and more difficult to move. You may feel sluggish. Again, motivate yourself to push through this. Expect highs, lows, and plateaus. If you keep adding reps and weight and striving to improve, you will. Again, it's a long and patient process. Take baby steps. Nothing grows in leaps however you will get the occasional surprise and achieve success that will motivate you even more. Keep trying and you will succeed just like I did! Realize the weight did not go on quickly so it won't come off quickly. Patience and persistence are the key methods. You can do it if you try. If I succeeded anyone can. I'm a regular guy that didn't like what I saw in the mirror so I did something about it. A body responds to these methods however you must implement them.

Start now. Remain motivated.

Music is an important part of my workout. I have many motivational songs recorded on my phone. They inspire me to work harder. Several times I've been about to take a break when suddenly an inspiring song comes on. Instead of taking a break, I move into the next routine or set of reps. Other songs have a certain portion that I work out to. When I ran on a treadmill years ago, I would program the fastest speed and highest slope for a certain portion of Van Halen's song, "5150". There were two guitar solos in there that were exactly one minute long. That set the expectation and resulted in me losing several pounds. I no longer run however music is always a part of my workout. I do pull one ear bud out on certain trails where cougars exist in case they sound a warning not to come too close. There are exceptions to every rule. I want some advanced warning before I dance with super kitty.

Music is an excellent motivator. It's very easy to obtain and store on a phone. No longer is a special device required. If ear buds don't work the speakers on most phones are now adequate enough for pleasurable listening. Use music to motivate you during workouts. A short time investment to obtain music will result in longer and more productive activity sessions. Computers also store and play music. Use all of these motivating factors to keep you incentivized.

Anger, denial, and frustration are all motivators. I can't tell you how many times I've broken off one of life's desirable tasks and worked out. Other times, I've had a down feeling and turned to my workout. Because my vocational work is mental versus physical, my work out helps circulate blood when I become numb in the brain from focusing too long. The rise in circulation would not occur had I remained in a seated position while performing my job.

Like a good sleep, activity can put a different perspective on things. We as humans tend to spiral in our thoughts to a point where they sometimes get out of proportion when we are frustrated. We speculate and imagine the worst. This is the wrong time to send that acid email. You can write it but don't send it. Instead, write it and then think about all angles and possible impacts it could cause during your workout. Disengaging from the thought process and performing an invigorating activity tends to lessen the impact of a less than desirable mental situation. It gives you time to think and investigate new scenarios. Often times, I have a totally different view of the situation after my workout. The once detrimental thoughts don't seem so bad after all. What seems important really isn't as much of a factor as I envisioned it to be. Life will and does go on. The frustration isn't the end of the world at the end of the workout like it appeared to be at the beginning. Use workouts to think things through. You will have much better rationale.

Denial hurts. There are no two ways about it. If you are denied by another then all that you are left with is you. This is a perfect time to exercise as it will boost your confidence. Accomplishing something is a better alternative to letting a situation eat away at you. Frustration results from the inability to change a situation. You can't change the thoughts of others. You can however use activity to move a dumb bell 50 times, produce endorphins that boost your happiness, and see a visual increase in physique size from the blood entering the muscle. Don't let the frustration of denial control you. Deter your thoughts away from that which you can't change to that which you can. Focus on you rather than changing the thoughts of another. Activity and the endorphins it produces can offset the disappointment of denial. Replace it with the pride of accomplishment, something that is within your control. Realize that a better body will attract a better partner. Invest in your future with exercise to minimize the effects of denial. Motivate yourself to become more appealing and you will face less denial.

The holidays have always been difficult for me as I have often been denied access to my children. During this weight loss effort, the holidays were very difficult. I got dumped the week before Thanksgiving. It was too late to change plans that were now vacant of my partner that I had looked forward to spending time with. I experienced the holidays alone again. My workouts helped to ease the pain and boredom. They gave me something to focus on. They set me apart. How many people do you know can claim they lost weight over the holidays? I did and I proudly announced it on Facebook much to the chagrin of others. So my holidays did have some good memories. Seeing the positive is the best motivator!

I've mentioned before that I've had a heart attack and I'm paralyzed. These are both motivating factors for me.

The heart attack left me with slight damage to my heart yet I could still perform the same amount of activity. I am fortunately under no restrictions. I also grew two new arteries each around two clogged ones. I was handed a new lease on life. I'm motivated to take advantage of that. I'm motivated to keep the blood flowing so it expands and strengthens these new arteries. My eating habits and exercise should reduce clogging by keeping my cholesterol at a more favorable level. My activity is expanding the quality of my life as well as extending my life. This is very motivational. I have some sort of control over my health that I failed to take advantage of in the past. I have choices available to me. Many don't. Why waste the gift?

Similarly, I paralyzed myself by lifting weights improperly. My right leg has less nerve control to it due to a ruptured disk in my back cutting off the messages by pressing on a nerve. As a result, my right leg tends to be weaker as there is less messaging to control the muscles. I use this to motivate me to work my right leg harder in order to strengthen it to the level of my left leg. I strengthen my leg on the benches at Red Rocks Amphitheatre. They are spaced farther apart than the stairs and thus require more lift in order to scale them. I do 10 steps with my right leg to 3 with my left leg. As a result, my right leg has improved in strength which improved my balance and posture. My right leg feels much stronger. Use setbacks in your health as motivators like I did. Use second chances to motivate you. The results may surprise you.

My good fortune motivates me. I'm over 50 and free of pain and restrictions. Some of my friends have damaged knees that limit their ability to hike and do stairs. Others have abused their bodies by smoking, doing drugs, and injecting things. I've done none of these and I'm pain free. I can push myself in areas where they can't. I've got this body that has given me so much. I use that to motivate me and give back to it by improving it in terms of looks and health. It would be a shame to have a healthy body and not use it. So many wish they had one. Celebrate your blessings by rewarding your body with health for giving you a pain free existence.

Several of my friends and family have diseases. Multiple Sclerosis is a prominent disease among middle aged women in Colorado. I've seen it limit several women by causing them to be fatigued to a point where they have to claim disability due to not being able to fulfill a full day's work activity. This limits their income too as disability only allows you to make a certain amount of additional earnings. In many ways MS stifles their entire lives. Similarly, diabetes limits my son's abilities as well as restricts his diet. The monitoring aspect of diabetes requires a time commitment thus robbing him of a fuller life. I learned from his diabetes and used it to my advantage in order to get my carb intake under control. For both diabetes and MS I treat them as motivating factors. Where others are restricted, I am not. If they can endure unwelcome pain, I can endure pain to better myself. Instead of sitting on the couch and wasting this gift of being pain free, I make the most of it by using my body while I still can. I live for the feeling of uninhibited lungs that I can expand to their fullest without experiencing the restricting of buildup. I celebrate not having pain and suffering and instead produce endorphins that make me feel even better. I'm so lucky to be pain free. So many wish they were. I can and will control my weight and physical appearance and level of fitness with mental motivation. If you have the power and are pain free, use your gift. It will prolong aging and you will feel so much better about yourself. Health is nothing to take for granted. It is to be celebrated and accelerated. Having pain free health is a great motivator.

Clothing can be a great motivator. Eventually you will get to a point where your existing clothes are loose while experiencing the joy of fitting into clothes from your past. I was able to again fit into my lettermen's jacket from high school. I also was able to wear a sweatshirt my mom had given me over 20 years ago. It was one of the last remaining things I had from her. Nothing beats the feeling of trying on the next smaller size and having that feel loose as well! It is so motivating! I lost several shirt sizes and ended up donating anything larger than a Medium. It was a pile of clothes three feet high! By buying the next smaller size, you sign up for keeping the weight off. I've had three events of buying new clothes since beginning my journey. In pants I went from 38" waist size, to 34" to a combination of 32" and 30". Similarly, I went to Medium and then Small shirt sizes totally skipping Large after originating at XL. Nothing speaks confidence more than a trim waist and a tight shirt that conforms to bulging muscles. Clothes are an excellent motivator for keeping the weight off. Once you achieve a size you can relax your efforts from loss mode to maintenance mode. If the clothes begin to feel tight, increase your activity until they are comfortable once more. Adjust your lifestyle from maintenance mode back to loss mode for a short period until you regain a level of comfort. If it worked the first time, it will work again and again. The clothes act as a boundary to keep you in check. NEVER go back to getting a higher size. That is an admission of defeat. Conquer my friend, conquer! Failure is NOT an option! If that attitude can bring a crippled space capsule safely back to earth, it can burn fat off.

Rewards are great motivators however they are typically an after effect. Still, it is a good idea to celebrate your success. I quit drinking beer at the beginning of my weight loss effort. After losing 20 pounds I went to celebrate with a nice cold beer as my reward. Although the beer was refreshing, it didn't bring the satisfaction I expected. My attitude and habits had changed to a point where beer wasn't as desirable as it once was. The taste wasn't there. My tastes had adapted to my new food group. I could feel the carbonation expanding my stomach. It was if I was tossing away a hard earned dollar when I drank that beer. When the bartender offered me a second one, I accepted it. I couldn't even finish it. That was the last beer I drank other than to taste a few sips while on a date. I haven't had a beer in over a year. I was beyond my desire for beer and fully into my new lifestyle. The temporary taste was not satisfying enough to offset the weight increases. As a result of eliminating beer, I was feeling great and loving it. What used to satisfy me now disgusted me. A lifestyle change like this is possible for anyone who persists. My new lifestyle is not a sentence, it's more of a refreshing and enjoyable experience where beer is no longer desirable to me. My tastes have changed. I have in a sense reduced the need to motivate myself not to drink. This requires less effort to motivate myself and thus makes my life easier by not having to try as hard as I once did.

Although changing my eating habits wasn't as hard as I thought, it did result in eating foods that were a bit mundane at first. Ironically, I never got tired of these foods and eventually my tastes adapted to a point where I craved them. I would eat bacon and eggs every day and enjoy it. I ate cheese sticks which were satisfying. I had meats such as ribs, chicken, and fish. I felt full and satisfied with these foods which was a motivator over the pain I had endured on my starvation diets. Eventually I got to a maintenance point where I loosened up a little. I have the occasional bun with my meat or once in a while enjoy a cookie. One way of motivating myself during this time was to satisfy the pleasures of taste by offsetting them with the visual satisfaction that I was in the mirror as I progressed.

I do limit my intake of wheat as much as possible. Between my friend Steve who has a great knowledge of foods and my son's Celiac disease, I avoid wheat. It has been genetically altered to a point where it permeates the digestive tract doing more harm than good. Even if that's not true, the thought of it is a motivating incentive that keeps me trim by avoiding wheat.

If I'm given chocolates, I have one now and save one for later. I always enjoy them for taste while avoiding using them for the satisfaction of feeling full and offsetting hunger. That way I eat less. I'm careful to make sure I keep the portions small. I don't want to expand my stomach. As a personal feeling, an expanded stomach tends to induce a feeling of hunger. Keeping it smaller reduces my hunger and therefore my intake. I get full quicker with a small stomach. This is another reason I avoid anything carbonated as it tends to expand my stomach. Wheat and starchy foods like bread, potatoes, and rice also expand my stomach so I avoid them.

I also balance my intake with the activity that I'm performing. I will recall that I've done aerobics for the last two days which should burn the excess intake. If not, I plan an activity to burn the calories I ingest. The knowledge that I will have to burn it off motivates me not to ingest it in the first place or at the very least, regulate my intake.

Pizza had the same effect as beer. I noticed it didn't satisfy me like it once did. I felt I was eating purely for taste and not getting filled up. I realized that pizza is one of those foods that keeps you eating yet never satisfies you. When I ate pizza I longed for my more filling protein based snacks such as cheese sticks.

In the same manner I that pizza no longer appeals, I no longer crave sugary foods. I avoid salty foods as they tend to cause you to maintain water which slows your weight loss. I drink only water, tea, and coffee. I avoid sugary or diet based drinks. My taste buds have adapted nicely. I get more taste out of the foods that I do eat as my tastes have acclimated to a point where they are no longer overwhelmed with excessive amounts of sugar and salt. Even dry lettuce tastes good to me.

I realized that our bodies can be reprogrammed to seek certain types of foods. I emphasize in this book that 90% of weight loss is mental however it's amazing how a certain way of thinking becomes a lifestyle where your body actually does the thinking for you. Note this point as being of extreme importance. A lifestyle change is not always climbing the same steep slope. As you transition, your confidence and thought processes start making it easier thus reducing the slope and amount of pushing you have to do in order to motivate yourself. It seems to get easier as your tastes change to match your menu. What a beautiful thing! It got easier for me to enjoy the foods that burned the fat off me while providing the protein to produce muscle. Again, being motivated adapted me to this new lifestyle and provided additional motivation by transitioning my desire from unproductive food groups to productive ones. At first I had to push myself mentally however my eating habits eventually became a natural part of my life. My transition had resulted in my tastes changing to a point where my body craved the good stuff.

Celebrating success through the occasional food treat is one way to motivate yourself. I have many other ways of celebrating and rewarding my achievements. I'll try a new hiking trail or new exercise. My rewards are mostly centered around things that have favorable results. When typing away at my computer starts getting to me, I start getting excited about exercising. I even lay awake sometimes envisioning exercise. I in a sense became fanatical and as with everything, I do have to provide some balance. More recently I've become accustomed to being fit and not as obsessed as I once was. There is a period of relaxation awaiting you as well. Earning it is not as difficult as you may think it is. Change your lifestyle. Incorporate fun activities and desirable yet satisfying foods. It will be difficult at first yet it will get easier as the motivation fuels itself as it did for me in these examples I have provided.

Hiking provides balance for me as I am able to combine social interaction if I go with a friend or date. The same goes with dancing. This new lifestyle allowed me to dance all night without fear of fatigue. I didn't have to worry about getting pulled over because I no longer drink. I was celebrating my success with something other than a routine workout. I was including desirable aerobic activities. Babes love a man who dances. All of this is very motivating for me. If I can dance all night there are fewer chances a man will have the opportunity to move in on my date. I'm enabling my fun by staying on the dance floor instead of sitting and watching others have the fun. That's motivational!

I close this chapter with a little story. A heavyset girl came to the weight loss boot camp. Before the evening meal, it was tradition to hike the mountain for a short burst of uphill aerobic activity. This girl came out and took several steps and then stopped.

She began crying and said, "I can't do it."

She had given up. She had let the ache of the fatigue control her instead of breaking through to the other side. Last I remember, I was an American, not an American't which means quitting is not an option. Don't give up, ever. The ache eventually subsides. Mentally prepare for it and break through to the other side. Persevere and enjoy the rewards motivation brings!

4. ACTIVITIES

The word exercise congers up the thought of tedious, sweaty, indoor hellish toil.. I prefer instead to be happily performing activities most of which are outdoor.

I prefer the word "Activities" over exercise. Although exercise is an enjoyable and rewarding experience for me, it's much easier to view it as an activity. Activity is a much more palatable word. Also, I know activity is a part of my new and exciting lifestyle where I experience life to its fullest. I plan my activities into my schedule as a "must do" rather than "I'll get to it if I can".

I was successful in my journey because I increased my activity level through a combination of activities that include hiking, climbing stairs, abdominal workouts, and weight lifting. I attained the level of weight loss and fitness that I am currently at by optimizing my routine through trial and error. I typically squeeze in two of these groups of activity a day when I can. I sometimes squeeze in all three. Before you read the next sentence, think about how much time you waste in front of the

TV and computer each day on meaningless tasks that yield little or no results. My routine takes me anywhere from an hour and a half to two and a half hours. It's really not that hard to find the time especially when you consider that commercials occupy up to twenty minutes of an hour long TV program.

I kept upping the activities as I surpassed goals. I now perform activities on an average of an hour a day. I do skip entire days. Other days I weave my activities into my schedule throughout the day.

One objective was to keep exercise low impact and injury free. Therefore I never ran a single step as it jars an already injured spine. I have had three very painful back incidents in my life. All were cured with horizontal bed rest for a period of two weeks. The last episode was 19 years ago. I've learned to avoid aggravating or furthering my back injuries by implementing low impact aerobic activities. I avoided surgery in the past and was glad I did. I rehabilitated my back by swimming and performing abdominal exercises. By applying what I learned from my past back incidents, I have been able to shape up without injuring myself during my new lifestyle.

Again, I can skip entire days and still lose weight, gain muscle, or maintain. Realize that this is a lifestyle change. If you can invest time daily in meaningless tasks, do you have the time available to improve your health, prolong your life, and avoid dying in a rest facility that reeks of urine? If you look at your schedule, I'm sure you can find the time. If you can't find the time, make the time. It's really not that hard. As I said, this has been a fun, hunger free journey for me. Plan to change your lifestyle and feel better. Implement the change. Enjoy life as it was meant to be with a sound mind and body.

My activity routines can be broken down into three groups:
- Weight lifting of dumb bells
- Aerobic activity
- Floor work

Of these three, I can break them down even further.
- Weight lifting of dumb bells (with some machine work)
  - Chest and arms (Triceps)
  - Shoulders
  - Back
- Aerobic activity
  - Hiking slopes

- Stair climbing
- Upper body
- Swimming (usually hotels, avoid club membership charges)
  - Floor work
    - Abdominal (abs) workout
    - Pushups

In the following paragraphs, I expand on these topics.

Weight lifting and dumb bells

Lifting weights burns fat while toning and building muscle. It also improves your strength and stamina. I have a love-hate relationship with weights. Mostly it's love. However there are some exercises I don't enjoy. They provide benefit so I continue to do them. On the other hand, some exercises have me raring to go. Chest presses give me a great feeling and really define my pectoral muscles (chest). They are fun and produce results. Excuse me for a sec, I gotta go pump out a few presses! Woo hoo!

The key to staying motivated is to do a combination of weight and repetitions that are doable. As you find your routine getting easier, increase the weight if you want bulk. Increase the repetitions if you want stamina. The main point is not to overdo it. Don't do a routine that leaves you exhausted or in pain. Don't set your expectations too high. Again, this is a method for a lifestyle change. The only way it will work is to have a routine that is pleasant. A dreaded routine will only result in you giving up and failing.

There are so many different weight training methods of exercise that I've heard over the years including:

- isolate the areas (back, chest, arms, shoulders),
- push-pull days,
- don't wait over 48 hours before working that area again, and
- if it's sore then rest it another day.

To me, all of these are fads except for isolating the area or particular muscle. That method works for me. My weight lifting routine is based on a dedicated group of muscles per day. I have days devoted to back, chest, and shoulders.

After my high school sports days, I never really got into leg exercises. I found that increasing leg size resulted in my pants not fitting correctly. Even though I don't work my legs much, apparently I work them enough. A woman recently told me that I had nice quads (thigh muscles). Her husband was once a punter in the NFL. To me, the compliment carried extra weight as she had complimented me on my achievement even though her past point of reference had achieved far more than I had.

I do however have to work on my legs in order to compensate for the slight paralysis in my spine. I climb stairs and also do squats on my Pilates machine. I combine this squat with my incline bench presses. I set the machine at an incline and push the sliding platform up with my legs while simultaneously pressing the dumb bells off my chest. This allows me to save time while performing two exercises at once. I have noticed some gains in my legs. My most noticeable gains are in my upper body where I concentrate the most.

In the past I had success with push-pull days. This is a method where one day is devoted to all push as in pushing the weight away from the body. The next day is all pulling towards the body. Pulling is difficult to achieve without machinery. I use the Pilates machine for rowing and pulling down. I do lack a good late pull down method.

I don't recommend any particular method of weight lifting yet I have learned from the fads as they passed through the gym. The culmination in this learning has resulted in success for me that I'm sharing with you. Again, trial and error work as does introducing new routines and changing things up every so often. Pick a method and try it. Give it three weeks. If it isn't working, find something that does. The point is to keep improving the process and its appeal. You are more likely to stick with it when the routine results in improvement. In the end, you will have an optimal routine like I do.

I started out with 15 pound dumbbells doing an entire routine (hitting every muscle group) each and every day with 50 reps per routine. I then increased to 100 reps. Eventually I broke the work out into three different muscle groups; chest, back, and shoulders. My success came by changing my routine and observing what works. I started with 50 repetitions and the 15 pound dumb bells. I then progressed to 100 repetitions per routine. Usually I did three sets of 50, 30, and then 20. I found I could do more reps in the first round and fewer as the muscle became fatigued. There are exceptions where I can do more. Let's just say that I stop when I realize I'm about to drop the weight on my head OR I am having to twist my body in a manner that is likely to cause injury as I try to squeeze out a few more reps.

As I desired to build muscle, I increased the weight to 20 pounds and reduced the repetitions to 50. Eventually, I took some of the exercises to 45 pounds where I try to do 50 reps of each. I haven't moved up in weight like the days of my youth however I really don't care. I've accomplished a defined physique with 45 pound dumb bells and I'm fine with my looks as well as my level of strength. I don't strive to continuously improve my strength as I don't want to force myself into injury.

The reason for the size of the weights I chose was simple: I chose what was available. The 15 pounders were given to me. I traded them for 20 pounders. I found 45 pounders for a decent price on Craigslist. I'm now looking for 60 pounders and 30 pounders however I'm going to keep the other weights. I'm not so much worried about increasing weight as I am improving strength. Besides, I'm on the other side of 50 where I heal slower and my joints are more susceptible to injury. Whereas weight lifting was an effort to constantly increase weight in my younger years, it's more of a gradual improvement nowadays with a focus on avoiding injury while still progressing muscle size and definition.

For me dumb bells are the best choice as they offer flexibility and don't take up much room. I can load them in the car or move them from the deck to inside based on the weather. I stash them under the end tables so they aren't in the way. A bench and long bar with removable weights is too bulky and space consuming for me. I do have a Pilates machine that was being thrown away. It fits nicely in the living room. I'll throw my couch out before I get rid of the Pilates machine. I keep my equipment to a minimum and try to maximize its use. I keep my equipment in the areas of my home where I spend my time. I don't restrict the equipment to a room that I visit infrequently as a reminder to keep working out. Find out what works for you based on your situation and limitations. Don't buy an expensive machine only to have it gather dust. Try it first and if you don't like it, use another method. Most machines have time limited return policies. Use them. Avoid machines that don't offer improvement. Don't let a machine sit unused. Find a way to incorporate the equipment that you have available into your routine.

My Pilates machine definitely improves my workout as it

offers the ability to incline my bench thus offering a variety of angles to do presses. This has enabled me to round my pectorals nicely. It also has introduced some pull exercises that I can't duplicate with dumbbells or free weights. Like it or not, an expensive (free for me) machine does have benefits that pay back nicely. Although I try to keep this lifestyle change free of charge, there are some investments that I have made and realized a huge return from. Still I took the frugal approach of finding second hand equipment.

I have listed various weight exercises that I do in a table below. They work for me. I'd suggest you try them, give them three weeks or so, and then reconsider their benefit based on the results you see. I have provided additional graphic photos and descriptions of each routine in the Appendix.

My Routine

- o Weight lifting of dumb bells (with some machine work)
  - Chest and arms (Triceps)
    - Presses at 6 different incline levels while squatting (45 lbs; 50 reps)
    - Presses at 3 different decline levels (45 lbs; 50 reps)
    - Flat presses (45 lbs; 50 reps)
    - Above the head arm extensions (20 lbs; 50 reps)
    - Level upper arm extensions (20 lbs; 50 reps)
    - Extending the arms on the Pilates machine

  - Shoulders (while wearing a weight belt for back support)
    - Behind the back presses (45 lbs; 50 reps)
    - Shrugs (45 lbs; 50 reps)
    - Upright rows (20 lbs; 50 reps)
    - Bent arm flies (20 lbs; 50 reps)
    - Extended arm flies (side) (20 lbs; 50 reps)
    - Extended arm flies (front) (20 lbs; 50 reps)

  - o Back
    - Rows on the Pilates machine (inclined)
    - Extended arm pull on the Pilates machine (flat, one chord removed)
    - Lat pull downs (side, inclined)
    - Lat pull downs (front, flat)
    - Bent over rows (45 lbs; 50 reps)
    - Single arm pull (45 lbs; 50 reps)
    - Standing back extension (45 lbs; 50 reps)
    - Horizontal back extension

- Aerobic Activity

  - o Hiking slopes
  - o Hiking trails
  - o Stair climbing
  - o Upper body
  - o Swimming (usually hotels, avoid club membership charges)

Aerobic activity is my chance to be outdoors and exercise my lungs. I've developed three areas I like, hiking, stair climbing, and upper body workouts. Hiking wasn't working until I introduced elevation changes which provided a low impact way of getting my breathing and heart rate up. This resulted in expanding my lungs to the fullest, one of the ultimate feelings a body can produce. My legs are also much stronger and have more stamina.

Hiking slopes worked the back of my legs. I had an excellent continuous slope right outside my door. It climbed 500 feet in elevation over 1.2 miles. Eventually, I could make it up and back in an hour. It was the perfect workout. One key learning was that it worked best for me to be ascending in the beginning and descending when returning. I did this slope just yesterday and was disappointed that it was downhill on the way back. My lungs wanted more challenge!

At first I had to stop a lot in order to catch my breath. As the summer progressed I went further and further. I would long for the occasional tree for shade in the summer and loath them for keeping the snow from melting in the winter. I did eventually conquer the slope without stopping. It took me about 25 minutes to ascend at the least. This is a perfect amount of activity for me. That applies to both the loss phase as well as the maintenance phase.

Another form of aerobic activity that I enjoy is hiking the stairs at Red Rocks. This effort was the second biggest producer of results as far as losing weight. Hiking was the first while weight lifting/abdominal repetitions were third. Again my success was due mostly to low impact elevation climbs at a steady pace versus running which jars the spine and aggravates my back injury.

Stair climbing allowed me to strengthen my thighs. Being paralyzed in my right leg from spinal nerve damage, I did 10 large steps with my right leg to every three for my left leg. One very important thing that kept me from injuring myself was to descend stairs without touching my heel, ever. Instead I would use the muscles to slow my descent standing somewhat tiptoed while mostly resting on the ball of the foot than lightly setting down. I never landed heavily on my heel. Again, low impact will preserve your body and avoid injury. That's why I don't jar my body by running. It's too impactful to my spine.

I'm always looking for an opportunity to expand my routine. This is America and opportunity is everywhere, including the areas where you exercise. While at Red Rocks, I observed others and saw several opportunities to do upper body and abdominals work. The results have been very positive. I use these routines for days I can't get to both aerobic and weight sets. Now they are a constant part of my visits to Red Rocks. The activities are profiled in the following paragraph and in detail in the Appendix.

I perform a number of upper body exercises. I do full body dips and extended leg dips. For the full body dips I'm up to 140 at 35 per visit to my little station. I visit four times as that's how many times I climb the stairs at Red Rocks where I ascend to the "dip station". I do 200 extended body dips in groups of 50 per visit to another area of the amphitheater. I found this was making my arms numb as I was working my triceps with a high degree of intensity. The blood was flowing to my triceps yet still they were numb causing me to have to shake my arms by my sides in an effort to offset the numbness by working the blood out. I decided to extend the triceps by doing curls so I do 100 curls per arm or 25 per visit (I just this week went to 50 per visit and 200 overall). The curls did two things, they offset the numbness created by the dips by stretching the triceps in the opposite direction. In addition, they gave me a method of building my biceps that didn't tax my tendons like the dumbbells did. My biceps stayed in the same plane with no side force pressure when doing curls. As a result, they have rounded nicely while my joints, tendons, and ligaments are pain and injury free. This "curl" exercise worked the bicep muscle while extending the tricep. The extension of the tricep soothed and eliminated the numbness that was caused by doing dips. For me, this is the perfect combination.

Whenever I have the opportunity to swim I take it. Usually it's in a hotel pool. I've yet to visit a health club to swim. Although I enjoy the act of swimming, I don't like having swimming as a regular part of my routine as it's time consuming and adds cost. My lifestyle change works best if my chosen activity is free of any cost. Swimming is time consuming as you have to change clothing twice. It also requires a facility to change and swim in. I am more of a spur of the moment type. Swimming did help rehabilitate my spine when I injured it due to improper weight lifting. Still, swimming has worked well in the past for me is an excellent form of shaping your entire body. That's why I partake if I can…but it's got to be a free side benefit. Lowering or eliminating cost is another motivation technique for keeping going as you transition your lifestyle.

Therefore, I avoid clubs as they charge to swim. If you have a free pool at your disposal use it. Apartments and homes are great places to swim. I haven't ever had the patience to maintain a pool so I don't have one.

Floor work

Floor work is my final method of exercise. Equipment that I use includes a yoga mat, towel, the Pilates machine, the occasional pillow and the occasional dumb bell(s). Floor work consists of:

o Abdominal (abs) workout
- 100 bicycles
- 100 toe touches
- 100 leg lifts
- 100 knees to the chest
- One of the following,
- 100 sit ups with one 45 pound dumb bells, or
- 50 sit ups two 45 pound dumb bells (taxes my joints in my arms more than my abdominals)
- 100 side twists on the Pilates platform
(can substitute Russian twists with a dumbbell)
- 100 side bends with a 45 pound dumb bell

o Pushups

Abdominal work has been a hit and miss effort in terms of success. At first I tried to avoid straight sit ups as the lever action often hurt my back until my core was strengthened enough to support the motion. Instead, I did crunches and various other exercises that tightened my core and curved my spine forward instead of leveraging from it. Doing these exercises straight on produced very little over the first five months. The side twists on the Pilates machine really made a huge difference as they caved in the sides of my stomach within two weeks' time after five months of trying.

Sit ups also helped flatten my stomach. After five months of core work, I was now able to do sit ups without arching and levering my back to the point of discomfort. At first I couldn't do eight sit ups. Now I can do 100 while holding a 45 pound dumb bell or 50 when holding two 45 pound dumb bells.

The final piece of the puzzle for rippled abdominals was leg raises. I once hated sit ups and leg raises. Now that I have a tight core, I crave them and approach them with vigor. They are fun and rewarding. I got my core in shape with the spine curving exercise thus levering my back was not as difficult nor as painful. This gradual transition worked for me while avoiding injuring my back further. The success I achieved for my abdominals took time and patience as well as trial and error. I was glad that I discovered an arrangement that makes abdominal workouts desirable.

Abs are amazing muscles. Once you get them cranked up they seem to be inexhaustible. Other parts hurt before your abs like the tops of your legs do in a sit up. Extending my legs so they are not bent as far at the knees solves this. I would highly advise that you push yourself in your core area (stomach area below the ribs and above the hips). I started working my core at the very beginning even when I was sporting a large beer belly. As my stomach declined, my range of motion increased. You will be amazed at how fast you progress in your ability to do repetitions. This is one area where I encourage you to push beyond pleasant. You will be glad you did as your progress begins to show. A strong core leads to better overall fitness. By having my core workouts on a separate schedule than weights and aerobics, I have achieved the best combination for me.

I was shadow boxing for about seven months with five pound dumb bells. My goal was to twist my love handles off. This never worked. I did see a slight decline in size but never eliminated the love handles. There wasn't enough horizontal force in pushing the dumbbells. The force was downward due to gravity which helped my triceps as my arm extended while doing little or nothing for my love handles even though I was twisting my torso. Like planks, I gave up shadow boxing. Neither worked for me. I do get the benefit of planks when I do pushups. Still, the core crunching, sit ups, and leg lifts created the best results.

Pushups work the chest, arms, and abs. By keeping your back straight during a pushup, you are in effect performing a plank as well. Abs are worked from the plank position which I hate and still hate. Although I can plank easier now that more core is in shape, I'm still uncomfortable in my lower back when doing pushups after about 25 repetitions. Planks have this effect on me too. I don't go beyond 25 repetitions in order not to tax my back. I tend to do my pushups facing downhill with my legs elevated on a chair or on the next bench seat up at Red Rocks. The elevation forces more weight towards your chest making for a better result. When I have dumbbells nearby, I used those to support myself during pushups as it is easier on my wrists then pushing flat off the ground. I use the hexagonal dumbbells as the round ones tend to roll whereas a flat side doesn't.

I do 100 pushups in increments. I never seem to get over a maximum of 50 repetitions per set with inclined pushups and again limit it to 25. I try to be methodical and slow during pushups while extending fully and touching my chest. Gone are the days of throwing myself in order to squeeze in a few more reps. I practise a steady positive thrust going up and a steady regulated resistance going down. Quality works as it avoids the potential for injury that striving for quantity brought with it. When I exhaust myself I break into smaller sets. Eventually I get to 100 even if I'm only doing ten reps per set (which is usually the case after 350 combined dips exhaust my triceps when I'm at Red Rocks).

Although having a workout partner sometimes helps to motivate you, most of these exercises I do alone. I've been able to convince the occasional friend to go to Red Rocks however no one really has a schedule and level of desire that matches mine. Hiking is a bit more appealing than my workouts are. I'm slowly adding hiking buddies now that winter is over. I drove myself to do these exercises throughout the winter and only caved on the coldest days. This level of dedication has proven worthwhile to me. I persisted even under some brutal conditions. I've been caught on mountainsides with lightening striking ahead and behind me. I've brought protection against cougars, encountered deer, and elk, and gotten drenched a couple of times. I've seen the leaves come and go, trudged through snow, fought the wind, and felt this discomfort of the hot sun. I wouldn't trade these experiences for anything. Twice in my life I have been outdoors during the changes in seasons. They are among the most memorable times in my life. How I survived 30 years in a cubicle I'll never know.

I am so fortunate to have seen what I've seen and experienced it in a pain free body. Life is so good for me. Won't you join me and share the happiness? Start changing your lifestyle right now. Celebrate your injury-free, sickness-free body while you still have it. So many bed ridden folks wish they could. Use the gift that you have been blessed with. I do and man am I happy. Change your lifestyle to include activities like I have. Make them fun and invigorating. You'll be glad you did.

5. EATING HABITS

I present what I ate (notice I didn't say diet) in order to give you an idea of how I was able to burn the fat from my body. I didn't restrict myself to a given menu. Instead, I changed my eating habits by focusing on protein and reducing carbohydrate intake. My menu was simple yet fulfilling. I ate low carb thus using my fat as a source of energy. I ate high in protein and put the protein to use by lifting weights and rebuilding muscle. I tried to avoid any and all processed foods in an effort to reduce the intake of unnatural compounds. This included wheat which has been genetically altered to a point where I believe it does more damage than good.

You won't believe what I ate in order to lose 60 pounds. Here's the list of the main diet:

- Eggs,
- Bacon,
- Cheese sticks,
- Chicken wings,
- Hamburgers,
- Chicken,
- Fish

As you can see, I was on a low carbohydrate (carb) diet. The important thing was that I was rarely hungry. I always felt full. There were maybe two days that I felt famished. Other than that, my mind was free of the pain of hunger which allowed me to focus on my life. Gone were the headaches and starvation I had experienced on my previous, fat free "diets". I wasn't distracted by food nor the hunger associated with it. This is very important if you are to succeed. My eating habits became a pleasant part of a changed lifestyle that was permanent. Therefore I avoided the roller coaster of weight gain and loss that typically accompanies most efforts in dieting.

This is a book about how I lost weight. It is not a book instructing you the methods for losing weight. Instruction to me is directive rather than inviting. If I tell you "what to do" rather than "how to do it" you will miss the key points. There are plenty of books out there that do that. I'm taking you on a journey that was successful for me and I hope will incentivize you to have the same body that I ended up with. I am sculpted and get many compliments. It has been an easy and fun journey. However, as with any exercise or eating plan, consult your doctor. Many doctors will tell you this form of protein based eating is unhealthy yet you can't argue with the success I've had in losing weight and curbing hunger. Therefore, I recommend that you pursue a few opinions and monitor your progress. The best way that I can recommend is to get frequent blood tests especially for health related indicators such as glucose and cholesterol.

That being said, I want to tell you what did and didn't work. Being anal and documenting my calories and carbs didn't work. Watching what I ate did. I focused on food groups rather than specific intake in terms of counting calories or carbs.

When I first started this routine, I read the Atkins diet. This diet uses a simple philosophy where you use your body fat as a source of energy instead ingesting your energy through carbs. You progress in two week periods of carb intake. The first two weeks you keep daily carb intake low and then slowly reintroduce them. It is a lot easier than you think mainly because I never felt hungry. The main thing to keep in mind is to eat protein and limit the carbs. This is very easy to do nowadays as labels have information on them labelling the carbohydrate content per serving. For instance, initially I thought I could drink milk however I saw the carb content was too high so I cut it out. I drank water, tea, and coffee throughout. My first week I averaged less than ten carbs a day. I still average less than 25 and I'm maintaining weight while building muscle. After your initial learning of carb content you can pretty much ditch monitoring your intake on a regular basis. You will have to moderate occasionally especially if you go to foods outside your core menu.

Here are some hints about carbs. I'll use pizza as an example. If I eat pizza, I'm never satisfied. It tends to make me hungrier. The dough tends to expand my stomach or at least gives me the feel it's expanding while fueling my hunger further instead of satisfying it. If I just eat the top layer and skip the crust, I feel full quicker. I've only had pizza three or four times in eight months and I don't miss it. The same with goes with beer. I thought that I would miss beer but I don't. When I hit a loss of 20 pounds I celebrated by having beer. First of all, it wasn't as satisfying as I thought it would be. The taste no longer appealed and the bloated feeling it gave me due to the carbonation expanding my stomach was unpleasant. The only pleasant thing about the beer was the fact that the beer was cold and it was a hot summer day. Honestly, I could get the same satisfaction of quenching my thirst from water. In fact, I drink a lot of water on this diet which really helps flush out the fat. It also guarantees I won't get a DUI if I stay out late listening to music.

The feeling I get when I eat carbs is none other than a feeling of bloating. This is especially true with beer. Most beers have carbonation added to them. This expands your stomach. For me, an expanding stomach feels empty. The result is a feeling of hunger that I have to feed. I'm going to go back to my high school football coach's statement about goal line defense. The best goal line defense is not to let the other team down near the goal line to begin with. That logic applies here. Don't create a problem and you won't have a problem to solve. Don't ingest anything carbonated and you will help curtail your hunger. In addition to beer, carbonated items include soda pop and seltzer water. Again, shrinking the size of your stomach is crucial. Bloating it with carbonation is counterproductive.

In the same manner I avoid carbonation I avoid sugar. Energy drinks are loaded with sugar. I get my energy from the fat I ingest and the mental attitude I have about working out. Now that I'm trim and my lungs are open, I have good blood flow and energy levels. I don't need to supplement with temporary energy from sugary sources.

I want to continue with the food portion of my eating habits. I'll address alcohol more in a separate chapter as alcohol consumption (or lack of) is very vital to your success.

Keeping up with your routine has a lot to do with how food makes you feel. Gravitate towards food that makes you feel full by satisfying your hunger while still keeping in mind that a body needs nutrition. There are so many diets and recommendations out there that I'm not going to go into detail about food and bore you with tasteless recipes that may have worked for someone but won't work for everyone. I don't like recipes as they are focused on a certain amount of intake. We are all different people so a recipe that fulfills one person might just leave another feeling hungry. Therefore, I eat what works for me to not feel hungry. This has been crucial to maintaining my chosen lifestyle. Again, I don't push recipes. Instead, I'm going to tell you eating habits that worked and how they worked for me.

Eating food that was high in protein and low in carbs was the key to my success. Proteins such as meat, cheese, and bacon have fat. I burned the fat and put the protein to use by building muscle. You must realize that these eating habits will work better for you if you are active, which I made fun and not feel like work. The combination of having fun and not being hungry made my lifestyle change enjoyable. I can't emphasize that enough. If you are taking in all of this protein, why not use it to build your body? If you aren't taking in carbs, why not burn your stored fat and the fat you ingest as energy through activity? It has been said so many times that diet and exercise (eating habits and activity) only work when practiced together. You will lose weight if you do one and not the other however it will come off slowly. By combining the two, you will lose weight faster and be more incentivized. Start planning your lifestyle change now for eating habits and activity then stick with it. I was successful at it. You can be. Keep optimizing the process until you find what works for you. Trial and error work. Find a way to be successful and happy.

I'm successful because I found the right combination for eating and activity. At an average weight loss of eight pounds per month, I'd say I was successful. Note however that there was a gradual decline in my weight loss over time as the slope of the graph becomes less. This is to be expected as your body adjusts to its new routine. Even though those last pounds take a while, they are the point when the most visual gain shines through. Also, I was still on a downward trend after starting to bulk up around the beginning of January when I increased the amount of dumb bell weight I was using. This is again proof that the combination I chose was working. You can't argue with success and I hope I'm getting you excited about your own weight loss journey.

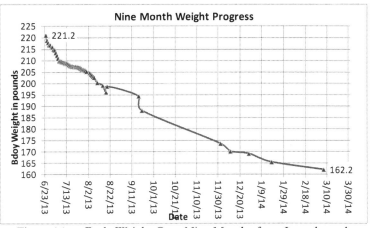

Figure 16   Body Weight Over Nine Months from June through March 2014

As my diet progressed, interesting things happened. My tastes changed. I noticed the taste of sugar and salt much more in my food and actually grew to dislike them. I liked the taste of the foods I was eating more and more. Although my menu was routine, I only grew tired of it on occasion. I would then eat something different. If the new food was carb based, I knew I would have to burn it off so I ate in a limited quantity while making sure I did some of my aerobic routine in order to offset the carbs. I would only have carb laden foods on occasion in order to add variety. I didn't want to reintroduce them permanently. I had worked so hard to get where I was. I wasn't going to go back to foods that left my unfulfilled without satisfying my hunger

Lowering carbs is really easy if you know what to look for. Avoid anything that is the color white such as bread, flour, rice, sugar, and milk. The exception is cheese sticks which kept me full and satisfied. I read that they are a great bedtime snack as they contain the sleep agent, melatonin. Regardless, they are a quick and easy snack that you can keep in the fridge or easily get at the grocery store prepared and ready to eat. I think Safeway caught onto my method of buying individual cheese sticks at a rate of $0.25 or less per ounce when they raised the price from 4 sticks for a dollar to 3 for a dollar. I think their computer showed an uptick in purchasing which they transferred into a price increase so I stopped buying them in individual form. Amazing how the price never went down after my volume of purchases did. My method of getting the best value now consists of comparing the sales and buying cheese packaged as sticks or in bulk in my effort to keep it below 25 cents per ounce.

Get used to having a plan for the foods that you will purchase before you walk into the grocery store. Go directly to the isles that contain your food choices, get your items, and leave. Try not to go hungry as the strategically placed items will lure you into buying food that will add weight. I remember when my son got diabetes and had to change his diet. Even at age four he could smell the sugar in the cereal aisle. Similarly, I recently went into Walmart's food section one day and stopped at the entrance. There in the middle aisle where the traffic entering the grocery section was heaviest, I was surrounded by carbs and foods enhanced with preservatives and chemicals to emphasize taste. I learned to power right by this strategically placed stuff and avoid it. I knew where my food was located and went directly to it. I'd suggest that you do the same so that you will be successful. They say that a marketing ploy used by grocery stores is to put the milk at the very back of the store. We often stop by for just a quart of milk as one of our regularly replaced items. The stores have caught on to this and place the milk at the back. The store marketing strategy is to place attractive items along the route to the back of the store where the milk is. By doing so, they're hoping to sucker you into impulse buying items you don't so much need as want. Don't fall for this. Have a plan to buy a targeted group of foods and get out without deviating. If you're going to deviate on anything, make it fruits, vegetables, or protein that offers good value and no preservatives.

The time of day that you eat has to work for you. I pace myself over the day and eat when I'm hungry. I eat individual items instead of full meals with variety such as meat mixed with veggie. I avoid potatoes eating them only as an occasional special treat. They expand my stomach making it feel hungry like bread and beer does. Being a bachelor makes this easier as I only have to prepare for myself and not a group of people. I also do all my cooking once or twice a week so that I don't waste time preparing food. I use the energy that heats the oven in a manner that maximizes efficiency. I take advantage of restaurant specials such as $1.25 ribs on Tuesday and $5.99 a dozen wings on Wednesday. I eat onsite and usually have leftovers. This gives me an opportunity to socialize and bring home premade meals that I can quickly heat up when I'm hungry. In some cases I don't even heat the leftovers up in order to save time. If I do cook, I'll put everything in the oven together and have enough for three to five days or even a week. Then I'll got out on the deck and work out or work outside on the computer while it cooks so I don't sit there and smell the aromas that make me hungry. I set my phone to go off as well as the oven timer so that I don't burn or overcook my meals. I shut the heat off and let the meal finish cooking with the residual heat. I only open the oven after it has cooled a bit.

When I finally hit a brick wall in weight loss and couldn't get to my six pack abs, I again turned to the internet for more information. I read that a six pack is about reducing your body fat to a point where your muscle is revealed rather than working your muscles to a point where they protrude to a level where you can see them. This made sense as I had been working my abs very hard for months without achieving a six pack. I had dramatically flattened my stomach and curved it in on the sides yet I wasn't seeing the muscles....(probably shaving my Yeti would have helped). I was doing up to 500 sit ups a day and 500 reps of other abdominal exercises yet it wasn't producing an obvious six pack. I read several diets for getting six packs and settled on one where I ate egg whites, tuna, and broccoli. Even with my determination I couldn't keep on this "diet" and went back to the more fulfilling one with oranges and bananas and nuts which I introduced in the seventh month of February 2014. I'm maintaining between 55 and 59 pounds lost but more importantly the increased weight of my dumb bells has really toned me to a point where I'm getting lots of compliments. The six pack continues to elude me but I'm happy with my body. I'm still fitting into size 30 inch waist pants. I still like the look of my abs in the mirror. Most importantly, I'm maintaining, not gaining. The six pack may forever be the car the dog chases but never catches. When you think about it, what's the dog going to do with the car when he does catch it? The same goes for me and six pack abs. The fun is in the pursuit! The key take away is that I prefer to not restrict my intake to point where I'm hungry and unsatisfied in an effort to pursue the look of a muscular six pack. In this continuous effort of trial and error, I had hit a limit. I'd gone outside my boundaries and created an unpleasant situation. Rather than gut it out and be unhappy, I chose to have a slightly ripped stomach and enjoy life while foregoing an obvious six pack. As a result, I've kept with my lifestyle change by reverting to a happier, more satisfying menu and eliminating hunger pains. This is the key to my own personal success. Trial and error is my best recommendation to you as well.

In closing realize that a lifestyle change usually requires you to change your eating habits in a manner that focusing on burning more than you take in. Or at the very least, burning as much as you take in if you are in the maintenance phase. Find a method that works for you and your metabolism. Resist snacking and fight the hunger temptation by replacing it with activity and satisfying eating habits that leave you feeling full. Fitness is directly related to your quality of nutrition. However, there is some trial and error in finding the combination that keeps you trim yet healthy.

6. ALCOHOL

I have totally quit alcohol on two occasions in my life. It is much easier than you think it is.

This next section needs to be read fully to the end because I recommend giving up alcohol and present a number of reasons why. So many people balk at this recommendation as I did for 35 years. However, giving it up was the best decision I ever made. Please read this entire section and see the benefits. I am the type of person that does not like to be preached to. Writing this chapter was difficult for me as it sounds like I'm preaching to you. If that is the case, so it shall be. I'm not going to miss this golden opportunity to improve your life and accelerate your weight loss effort. I'd rather go back on my principals a bit to provide you with potential benefits.

I did a lot of research on the web to get where I am. Of course there is a stigma about the accuracy of information on the web. Be careful what you read and implement. I will share my personal success by telling you that the information on beer guts was very helpful. At one point I read that beer and alcohol in general enlarges your liver. I knew that shrinking my liver would reduce my stomach and more importantly reduce my waist. Again, major motivator for me was a flat, muscular stomach. Still, I didn't give up alcohol entirely until October after starting in June. At that point I was down 35 pounds. Once I gave up alcohol, I dropped nearly 25 more pounds. There were other benefits as well that I will present in this chapter. First I want to establish the time line and my phases of success as I limited and then eliminated alcohol.

I quit drinking beer when I started this weight loss effort on June 26, 2013. I still craved an alcohol buzz so I researched a replacement for beer. I read that hard liquor was void of carbs. I moved to a combination of bourbon and water and started seeing success as my weight was declining. I could still taste sugar in the whiskey yet I was losing weight. I was happy with my progress and the fact that I didn't have to give up my one vice in life. Then one night I went to a Halloween party with my girlfriend. We had a spat and I drank too much. She had warned me that I had few chances to keep her. Luckily she gave me another chance after I pleaded and told her the alcohol was part of the problem. I had gotten so drunk that I was hung over for two solid days. I had to film two Doritos commercials for the Super Bowl contest the day after the party. I was miserably hung over the whole day. It had been quite an effort to coordinate the cameraman and actresses for the commercials so I couldn't back out and wait until my hangover cleared. The messages of being hung over and almost losing a relationship were very clear, it was time to quit alcohol especially if I wanted to keep my relationship. I had previously quit alcohol for my second wife and knew I could do it to save my current relationship. Even though I am no longer dating the girl I quit for this time around, I've kept my promise to her as I am a man who greatly values integrity and sticking to my word regardless of whether someone is present in my life or not. I have adopted the promise not to drink for my own personal wellbeing. I've had one whiskey and water on Thanksgiving weekend and two Jello shots plus a Fireball shot at a Super Bowl party. Both times it felt like alcohol was poison in my body. Frankly, I don't miss it at all. My life has improved dramatically due to this decision.

Losing alcohol was the best thing I ever did. At age 52, I could still party like the college days. I was being stupid as I was risking a DUI and had been for 35 years. My number was up and I knew it. By quitting drinking I could now be the designated driver for my date. More importantly, I can stay until the last song when I am out listening to live music, one of my favorite things to do. I can drive home at 2 AM and have no worries about getting pulled over. When I drank, it was always a game of cat and mouse. If I had ever been caught, I would have been in trouble even though I gauged my intake in an effort to be below the legal limit. The laws are so stringent these days, quitting was my only option. The "one beer" no longer makes you legal especially when you consider the wrong cologne can raise you to a level of 0.03. With most laws starting at 0.05, there isn't enough head room for just one beer. The only solution for me was to keep alcohol entirely out of my system.

A DUI ruins your life, period. If you have never had one, read this paragraph and understand the consequences. Fortunately I never had a DUI. Most of this information comes from having watched others suffer through it. A DUI costs a minimum of $10,000 and upwards of $100,000. A cab will cost you $40. Sure you have the inconvenience of going to get your car in the morning and perhaps having it towed, stolen, or broken into. These inconveniences pale in comparison to a DUI. With a DUI you have to check in daily to see if you have to go take a breathalyzer. In the state of Colorado where I live, the court will assign you a random color. When you call in to check for your daily test, you must go in and take a breathalyzer test if your color is the color on that particular day. These tests are random and made to catch offenders. They are a regular hassle that you simply don't need in your life especially if you don't have a license and need to find a way to get to the testing sight. Losing your license means bumming rides, coordinating with public transportation, hoofing it or riding a bike (the last two are affected by weather), or driving yourself and risking getting caught. None of these options are desirable. Several aren't worth the risk of getting further charges levied against you. Driving without a license and/or a DUI can land you in jail. It's better to walk home and sober up than it is to walk to a test facility every day. Another more sensible option is to get a room which is only $50-$100 versus thousands in lawyer's fees, insurance rates, and lost productivity that all come with a DUI.

The DUI random checkup tests themselves have a fee thus adding additional cost. Worse yet, you have to arrange your more distant travel so that you can test in your destination city if your color comes up. Some private facilities will set you back fifty dollars to do a test when you are on the road. In addition to arranging testing, you may have to get permission to leave the state until your trial occurs. Even if you don't spend time in jail, which is highly unlikely, you are out on bail contingent on your abiding by the rules. One rule usually requires you to stay local to your court district or state. Again you have to get permission to travel and arrange to test at your destination. So think about what this involves. In order to travel, you have to get permission in advance from the judge to leave the state. If you have a lawyer, you will be paying them to petition the judge in addition to having to perform all of these arrangements in advance of your trip.

Another hassle associated with getting a DUI is the limitations it can place on your driving. If you are required to install a breathalyzer, you will incur costs and your driving ability will be limited to using only vehicles that have breathalyzers in them. If you get caught in a vehicle without a breathalyzer, you face additional charges and loss of your limited driving privilege. Note that driving is a privilege and not a right. It can easily be taken from you. Breathalyzers are hassles in other ways. They sometimes require a random test when you are driving. At other times, they can fail and leave you stranded. On occasion, they can produce false readings. The readings are monitored and there is a charge for them.

Breathalyzers are also embarrassing. One time I was in a parking lot in my pickup next to a car that was lower than me. I saw the driver duck over and naturally was curious. I realized that he was breathing into his breathalyzer in order to start his car. He was so embarrassed by it that he would duck down when performing his test. I was grateful to have avoided similar embarrassment.

As you can see, DUI's are one huge hassle that you don't need. Stopping drinking avoids them. Aside from the hassle, there is the safety factor. Driving impaired risks you and everyone else on the road. Wouldn't it be better if our police forces were pursuing criminals and solving crimes rather than babysitting roads to catch DUI offenders? It would lower your taxes if we had less police officers dedicated to DUI patrol. Yet another benefit of quitting.

I'll get off my soap box about DUI. However, there are so many more benefits to quitting drinking that I have personally realized. Number one is I save money. At five bucks a drink, two to four drinks a night, four weekends per month, the cost can easily reach $160 per month. That's half a car payment folks. And you usually tip 20% on top of that.

In addition to cost, quitting alcohol is good in other ways. You lose weight faster when you stop drinking and you are more likely to keep on your exercise and eating routines. I've "heard" that alcohol restricts weight loss. I have proof that it did in my case. I lost eight more pounds in three weeks after quitting entirely. I was amazed and remarked to my girlfriend that I was still losing at the same rate while keeping my routine the same. I was at a total loss of 43 pounds at this point and was amazed that I hadn't yet reached a plateau. She noted that I had quit drinking. I realized what that meant to my weight loss progress. By not being hung over the next day, I was less likely to duck workouts due to fatigue. Don't get me wrong, I've burned off many hangovers with a workout. However, it was a painful process that took extra incentive. The ONLY way these weight loss methods that I am presenting will work is to make them pleasant and without pain. So why add the pain of suffering through a hangover? This book is about a lifestyle change that is supposed to be fun and rewarding. Like anything there is effort involved. Quitting drinking makes that effort easier. I also noticed that I was more likely to workout evenings if I didn't have that happy hour drink that made me sleepier. My sexual abilities improved and I could dance all night. I was dancing more and enjoying it. Dancing turned nights out into aerobic activity that further burned weight. I was having so much fun without alcohol that I didn't miss it. Final benefits include: I could remember the night before and was making more rational decisions. Alcohol caused my mind to go through a series of highs and lows. I was now much more consistent mentally. As a result, I was much happier. That in itself was making me much more attractive.

If I can quit alcohol anyone can. There were factors in my life that pushed me towards alcohol. I have high cholesterol which alcohol supposedly helps lower. I came from a family with an alcoholic father. There were many embarrassing times growing up as the son of the town drunk. These included financial embarrassment. While other families vacationed at destinations, I worried about a place to live, having food, and having decent clothing. A family member on my father's side was tested and told me that she has a gene that is common in alcoholics. I most likely have that gene too although I've never been tested for it. I'd have a tendency to crave alcohol based on this genetic condition. By quitting entirely as a lifestyle decision, I'm less likely to cave into my cravings. Quitting was made easier by having a stronger desire to be fit than to catch an occasional buzz. Alcohol is a depressant. My happiness has increased without it.

Alcohol may have offset my high cholesterol as a small side

benefit. My father's side of the family has a liver disorder that keeps our cholesterol at 450. Furthermore it keeps the "bad" cholesterol high and the good cholesterol low. People freak out when their cholesterol is 200 or above. Mine was twice that plus. Most men in my family die in their 50's due to cardiac issues. I myself have had two blocked arteries and a heart attack that resulted from the blockages. Luckily I had a natural two way bypass where I grew two arteries around each blocked arteries. I never knew that was possible however this undeserved gift has been a motivator in my effort to better health. Although alcohol may have offset cholesterol production in my body, I believe my new lifestyle improves it even more.

Getting back to alcohol, it's easy to see why I would seek alcohol to offset my cholesterol (if the rumor that alcohol lowers cholesterol were true) and possible genetic craving. I quit in favor of enjoying life more. Quitting wasn't hard. I overcame my desires in pursuit of a happier life. I look and feel so much better. You can quit too if you so desire. Put your mind to it as a part of your lifestyle change. My looks improved too. My face is not as puffy and I don't have bags under my eyes.

I believe quitting alcohol shrunk my liver. There are several indicators of this. As you can see from my pictures, I had a rather large beer gut. Now that I've lost it, I have somewhat of a shelf where my rib cage drops off to my flat and toned stomach. Because my liver

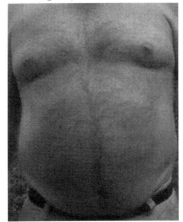

Figure 18 Before I Had a Beer Gut

resides under my rib cage, I believe that it expanded my rib cage to a point that created this shelf when my liver shrunk and my rib cage remained in the position that once accommodated my

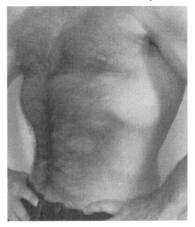

Figure 17 After I Was Near Six Pack Abs

larger liver. Inflammation is the body's way of telling you something is wrong. When you twist an ankle it swells. My liver was swelled. I believe it was trying to tell me something. I shrunk it and the swelling ended. I shrunk it by eliminating alcohol. I'd rather look better than catch a buzz. I'd rather not have a swollen liver. If you drink, I'd highly suggest that you consider quitting. I did and I'm happy I did. Note that my internet investigation initially stated that alcohol enlarges your liver and gives you a beer gut. This was my incentive for quitting. I don't truly know if my liver shrunk or my stomach became more muscular. I do know that I went from spilling over 38" pants to comfortably wearing a 30" waist. That is proof enough for me.

In closing I would like to restate that I'm living proof there are many benefits to eliminating alcohol consumption entirely. At the very least, note what worked for me in terms of losing weight. Cutting out the beer resulted in a loss of 35 pounds. Quitting alcohol entirely resulted in losing 25 more pounds and having a flat stomach. I prefer that over a temporary buzz any day. I'm not out to ruin the party however I would be very proud to improve or even save a life by convincing another the benefits of eliminating alcohol.

7. WORK HARD, PLAY HARD, STAY HARD

My Theme for the Last 20 Years. Been There, Done That, Bought the Tshirt
(Actually I sell a Tshirt at this website: http://www.cafepress.com/stayhard)

I am not a muscle head who is pushing a fad that goes around a gym. I am an average man that turned his body from flabby to hard. I am writing a book to help you do the same as easily as possible whether you are a man or a woman, young or old. I'm not trying to push the ultimate workout on you. I'm offering to get you an easy way to get trim and proud. No, scratch that. I'm offering you methods to implement a better lifestyle of happiness and fitness.

I need to interject a paragraph or two as to why a lifestyle is so important. A lifestyle projects your image to people. If you don't believe me, read the singles ads and posts. See what people are looking for. Also see what rejects you from the post. I did this and a common denominator surfaced. Woman like active men who are not couch potatoes. Women also sound terrific until you get to the point where it says BBW which stands for big, beautiful, woman. For me, this and smoking were reasons to exit stage left when I perused dating profiles. Within this book I solve both of those problems. I provide men a way to become fit and active as well as taking the "big" out of BBW.

Staying active is not always the fault of one's personal mental drive. Sometimes there is a root problem. Such is the case with low testosterone. In his book titled "Man 2.0: Engineering the Alpha", John "Roman" Romaniello talks about how his life improves when he doubles his low testosterone.

John wrote, "Over the course of the next several months, I dove into all the literature I could find and started making a lifestyle overhaul. I doubled my intake of saturated fat. I used high doses of fish oil. I cut carbohydrate intake to virtually 0 for close to two months. I was draconian about the times I went to bed and woke up. My sex drive returned rather rapidly. In 6 weeks, I felt different. After 12, I got tested again, and my testosterone levels had literally doubled–doubled! I was productive again. I started dating. I reclaimed my physique and liked the way I looked again. I felt alive again."

Does this sound familiar? Lifestyle overhaul? Low carbs? Saturated fat intake? These are the very principals that changed my life. I haven't promoted the fat as much as protein however it is an essential part of my menu. The point is, the solution for virility might be just around the corner in the form of these changes I recommend. It wasn't just me, a 52 year old man that realized a difference. A man in his 20's did as well. These improvements were a result of the very same method's I'm suggesting that you try in your quest to improve. Try these methods and see if they get you off the couch and into a happier lifestyle. If you are a couple, try them together. Nothing in this book limits you to an individual effort.

As far as solving the BBW (Big Beautiful Woman) issue, again, use the methods in this book. Beauty is not limited to looks, this I know. Internal beauty is a wonderful attribute in a woman. However, big as in overweight is a turn off for most men. I'm not putting heavier women down here, I'm stating a fact as to how men perceive you. These methods I preach can help your get rid of the big and bring out the beautiful on the outside. So many internally beautiful women don't get noticed due to our emphasis on external beauty. Even the loss of some weight can make you more attractive and happier to a point where your inner beauty becomes more obvious. Once you get fit and start feeling better about yourself you will be much happier. This will go a long way towards improving both your inner as well as outer beauty. You will carry yourself with much more grace and smile more than grimace. Happiness is attractive. Grouchiness and pudgy is not. Been there, done that. When you improve your level of fitness, you will seek looks from men rather than hide due to your embarrassment about your size. Your clothes will fit and feel better. As a human with the power to take control of your life, you have the ability to pursue happiness. It won't take as much effort as you think. It can be more fun than you think. Set your mind on the goal not the effort. Then make the effort fun, enjoyable, and doable by changing your eating habits and incorporating activities into your life. Transform your lifestyle so that you can realize the same success that I did. I became more fit and much happier. I'm not made of anything different than you are. I just got fed up one day and implemented change. Try it yourself. You are perfectly capable.

I thought about naming this book "Work Hard, Play Hard, Stay Hard". Instead I chose to name this chapter with that title because it has relevance to a more specific subject. This phrase supports my theme for successful fitness. In order to get fit and maintain fitness, there has to be a balance between work, play, and the fitness effort. If there isn't, you will go insane from trying too hard or give up altogether from trying to do the impossible. My methods aren't impossible, they're enjoyable. If they weren't, I couldn't employ and maintain this lifestyle change I've been continuously telling you is the key to your own success.

I'll shed a little light on how this "Work Hard, Play Hard, Stay Hard" theme worked during this period of weight loss for me. Like anybody these days, I was living a normal life with normal commitments in terms of work, relationships, and most importantly; available free time. I wasn't living luxuriously, I was living my way. It was a bit difficult as the six figure career that I had expertise in was no longer available to me. Instead, I was launching a startup on a budget and struggling. Still I was living on a mountainside in the Rockies near a town that had live music five nights a week. Although I was only renting a room versus owning a home, I was living in paradise. I had found a situation that worked for me and gave me happiness in addition to the ability to transition to my new lifestyle. Like my fitness effort, I didn't wait for the financial improvements to come. Instead I made it happen based on the situation as it was. If you wait, it will never come. You will always be promising yourself that you'll get to it without actually getting to it. If you act now, you can have it. This is a key success to a lifestyle change; act now regardless of your situation. Mine was about as dire as it had ever been. That would have been a good excuse to wait for a better time to lose weight. There is no waiting needed. There is only a time to make a decision and begin your new lifestyle.

I worked hard and played hard. In the process, I got hard.

While growing my business, I worked as hard as I wanted to, not as hard as someone else wanted me to. As a business owner, I was in control of my life. I wasn't so much working harder as smarter. I was promoting a new technology that could improve wireless speeds to 1,000 faster than the current rate. Still, it was hard convincing companies that you had a technology that would change the world immensely. I had the same road blocks as everyone. I have the same road blocks with this book especially when one considers the fact that successful books rarely come from every day Joe's. Instead they come from muscle heads with fitness degrees that provide a false front for a product they are pushing. I didn't have any of this backing or momentum working in my favor. I had to implement my lifestyle changes in my situation as it existed. I couldn't wait any longer for things to change. I had to take on this task along with the other tasks in my life. I'm no different than anyone else. The world doesn't stop turning in order to give us a break. We have to take things in stride. The lifestyle change begins when you decide it does.

I always thought that I had to be an employee. Looking back I realized that situation was controlling my life. I felt the best position for me was to be independent and contribute at my chosen level versus a level that was dictated to me in an annual review. The annual review usually resulted in a raise that was below the increase in the cost of living. Thus, I was losing money. I wanted to live in the Rockies and work from home. I chose to start a business that enabled me to do this. Changing my commute from an average of fifteen miles to six feet helped a lot as did making my schedule flexible to a point where I worked and played according to my decision, not a nine to five commitment. When I got burned out, I took a hike and rejuvenated. I planned my day around the weather. In Colorado we get afternoon thunder storms so I'd hike or work out on the deck in the morning in the sun and work on the computer in the afternoon when it rained. Evenings and Sunday afternoons were left to my pursuit of live music. Life was good. I had made a transition to a lifestyle that enabled happiness in more areas than just my health. This is very important in your overall lifestyle change in addition to the changes in activity and eating habits that I recommend. I did tackle a number of changes at once which in some instances can be detrimental. Realize that setting myself towards a new lifestyle resulted in the various changes complementing each other in a manner that resulted in progress as well as a much happier life. If you yourself are miserable, consider some of the changes I made. Again it's about happiness on the journey rather than a destination. If you wait, it may never come.

Playing hard went from anchoring a bar stool to weight lifting on the deck and climbing elevations. I also began to experience the many hiking trails that surround the town I live in. To me this was play. I listened to music, was outside in the sunshine, and was enjoying the beautiful scenery of Colorado. All of the while I was accomplishing the final step, stay hard. I was going from Mr. Softy to semi ripped definition. I wouldn't win any contests but I was turning heads and getting compliments on my body. Both of these were motivational factors that kept me going. More importantly, I was now very happy. As a result my life became a rich experience of human interaction and joy. It was not a miserable journey of sweat and starvation. I had found the key combination that made my lifestyle change enjoyable.

Staying hard means keeping my muscular definition. I'm down to working the major muscle groups once a week. I spend a day on my chest and arms, one on my shoulders, and one on my back. These are intermingled with my abdominal and aerobic activities. This combination of muscle building and aerobic activity has allowed me to maintain my pant size as well as my muscle definition. As with anyone, I could always work harder and pursue bigger size. I don't do this as I am happy with where I'm at. I feel good after my workouts. I don't over do it now that I have trimmed down. I eased up a bit and let other things into my life. If I start feeling like I've gained weight, I will up the activity and restrict my foods a little. I know now that I must keep somewhat of a vigil or risk gaining it all back. I've come so far that I need to keep a happy balance while realizing that sometimes it may not come as easy as others. That's ok now that I've achieved a level.

This combination of work hard, play hard, and stay hard is now working wonders for me. Find your own combination by employing these simple methods for your lifestyle change. You will be much happier in the end.

8. HITTING A PLATEAU

You will eventually hit a plateau with any fitness effort. It is unavoidable. It can happen in your weight loss, muscle growth, or just in the number of repetitions or the amount of weight you can handle. You are human and you eventually reach your capacity. It happens. There are positive ways to deal with it

Three things can happen when you hit a plateau. You can find a way to increase your progress, you can remain at the same level, or even you may even digress. It all depends on you. There is nothing wrong with a plateau especially if you are happy where you are at like I am a year after starting my journey. There are however ways to improve once you hit a plateau and I will discuss these in this chapter. I've hit plateaus several times. For the most part I've maintained. In some areas, I've improved. Luckily, I've yet to digress.

My first plateau was in my stomach area. No matter how many abdominal repetitions I did, I couldn't get my abs to reduce to a level where I was happy nor could I get to a six pack. I had read on the Internet that a woman had success with boxing twists improving her stomach. I tried trunk twists for months to no avail even though I was holding dumbbells while doing it. There wasn't enough lateral force from the dumbbells. The main force was downwards due to gravity. I knew that I needed to have a lateral force on my stomach in order to tighten up the side areas. This could have easily been accomplished with a piece of stretch rubber and a stationary object such as a couch or a pole. Lacking those I waited. When I heard that a friend was throwing out a Pilates machine, I saw it as an opportunity to solve my problem. This device uses a pulley setup to move you on a sliding platform. You can incline the platform and increase the resistance. These side twists helped me to get over my plateau and cave in the sides of my stomach.

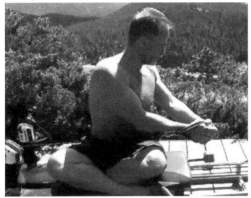

Figure 19 Side Twists on the Pilates Machine Were Key to Flattening My Stomach

Within two weeks of having this device I started to see definition in my stomach. My abdomen went from convex to concave. It was a welcome solution. The side twists bore results almost immediately. The friend who gave me the machine encountered me after I had been using if for a month.

Her first comment was, "You look good!"

Of course I was glad to hear that.

My second plateau resulted in my frustration in trying to reduce my love handles. The "muffin top" didn't seem to leave my sides no matter how many boxer twists I did. Frustrated, I turned to the Internet where I discovered side bends. These exercises are done while holding a dumbbell adjacent to my hip and bending down sideways fully one way. I then lift up sideways the other direction. These took the muffin top down in two days after trying for almost eight months. That was the fastest improvement I ever saw throughout all of my journey.

I'm not so concerned about hitting a plateau with my weight but then again, I never thought that I'd be near my high school football playing weight of 158 pounds (I made it down to 162 pounds). As I have mentioned previously, I currently judge my current weight in the mirror and with how my clothes fit rather than with the scale. I stopped measuring after I felt I had hit a plateau. Instead of focusing on losing more, I focused on maintaining.

Eating habits can also hit a plateau. With so many unhealthy foods to lure us, sticking to your lifestyle foods can be difficult. This is especially true when at parties

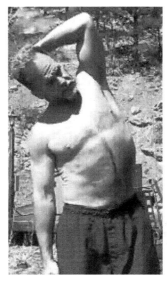

Figure 20 Side Bends Took Away the Love Handles in Two Days After Months of Trying

or during the holidays. My advice in this area is simple, be good as often as you can. You are going to cheat eventually or occasionally, it's a fact. Remember that the weight didn't go on or come off quickly. As long as your average intake is healthy, occasional spikes should not bother you. In fact some weight loss methods I discovered recommended binge eating in order to reset your body from starvation mode. This tendency towards starvation is a way the body protects you by hoarding calories in an effort to get you through lean periods. It's a mode that creates a plateau of sorts where you don't seem to be losing weight no matter what you do. If this happens, try to avoid starving yourself and instead increase your activity and eat normally. If your body is getting plenty and burns most of it off, it won't tend to store food as much as if you starve it. Again, it's all trial and error. Learn what works for you. My toleration period is three weeks. If I don't see a change in three weeks, I try something new. This works in terms of food intake and the starvation mode. Change the balance in your activity and eating in order to get back on the weight loss track. Experiment. Work through the plateaus or accept them if you are in a desirable state according to your metrics.

I have hit a plateau with my desire to improve muscle size. I know now I have to change something in order to improve. I'm looking at several new activities to try including a new method known as TRX. This method uses suspended straps with handles to perform a variety of exercises. One area I'm lacking in is a lat (lateral muscles in the back) pull down machine. I'm not strong enough to do lat pull ups with the weight of my entire body. Therefore I need to get a machine or routine that enables me to pull and develop my lats. I'm hoping TRX brings this opportunity for improving my upper back and lats. I also want to try paddle boarding and canoeing. Both are fun outdoor activities that beat rowing in a gym. I'll save indoor rowing for the winter months while trying outdoor rowing on water in the summer or perhaps in Arizona.

Life in general hits a plateau. There are limits associated with the time of year. For instance, certain fruits and vegetables are seasonal. I found this out when oranges got scarce (and as expected, the price increased). Strawberries and peaches also are available only certain times of the year. This variation in availability requires that you be flexible with your food choices. Always have alternatives available to avoid just buying junk when healthy foods get scarce. I haven't gotten into buying frozen fruits and vegetables however some people have found it to be a very successful and more economical alternative to fresh fruits. Again, find what works for you through trial and error.

The weather changes with the seasons and causes plateaus by limiting the activities you do. This didn't happen much to me because I'd go shirtless on sunny days even when it's 40 degrees out. But then again, I live in Colorado where the weather is dry and the sunshine is plentiful for the most part. I don't think I could have done this on the more humid east coast nor

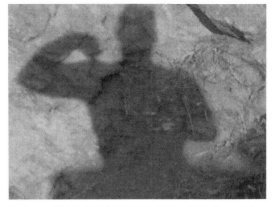

Figure 21 My Shadow Tells Me a Lot About My Progress

could I have lived through the 20 degree days. I did put on a ski jacket and gloves in order to hike both the mountain and Red

Rocks on some fairly cold days. I even trudged through snow about six inches deep or had to hold the hand rails when descending icy steps at Red Rocks. I overcame these minor inhibitors and stuck with my routine. Nothing was going to keep me from being fit. If I can do it, you can too. Plateaus in the weather break eventually. Plan for them and get through them as best you can. My activities allow me to remain warm while conducting them. My chosen place to live allows me to change elevation in order to find a suitable temperature for conducting my activity. Look for these various opportunities to offset plateaus.

Expect to hit plateaus and even valleys as you progress be prepared for them. Try different methods to overcome them. Eventually your gains will become incremental but they'll still be gains. That will keep you improving. If not, get to a plateau where you are happy and maintain. Avoid digressing at all costs. You've come too far to go backwards now.

9. AGING AND OTHER DISCOVERIES

I discovered a lot about myself on this journey. Some of these discoveries will benefit the younger crowd that reads this book. As I mentioned, I do target the subject of getting fit for males above 50. I have a summary of my transition for the above 50 readers as well.

Like anyone, I thought age 50 was old and decrepit up until I was in my 30's. I would never have thought back then that I could accomplish what I do now on a daily basis. At age 52 I don't feel any different than I did back then. Some of my friends describe themselves as slowing down. My only noticeable differences is that I don't lift as much weight and my tendons get sore much quicker. My muscular abilities and stamina seem to be related to the effort I put into improving them. I don't feel any limits as I power through my workouts like I did in my younger years.

I've noticed that aging appears mostly in my skin in the areas that are exposed to the sun. For me this is my face and my hands. Other than that, my skin does not seem to be aging much. Even in the areas where I have lost a lot of weight, my skin has tightened up. I don't have sagging or wrinkles. Two realizations come out of this. First, it's true what they say about the sun. It will age you. Second, your skin does respond above age 50. It is still elastic and flexible. I believe that by avoiding smoking, my skin stayed healthy and much more adaptable to my size.

I had a fear that my muscle size was never going to be what it was when I was younger. I had heard that men's muscles begin to shrink after age 40. I have proven that wrong. I'm as muscular as I ever was. I would have never thought that at age 50 and above. I'm proof that you can realize muscle gain.

I wrote in the Forward how my attitude has changed as I have written this book over the last several months. I went from being vain about my appearance to being happy with my health. Most of this was due to having a wonderful woman come into my life. She has become a close friend who has increased my happiness. She is beneficial to my journey as she too maintains a healthy and active lifestyle. We have many interests that are in common including hiking and the foods we eat. We share a lot of fruits and protein based foods while avoiding processed items. She has been very good for my lifestyle change. She has shown me how to be more happy with my inner self than my outer appearance. She is a result that I never imagined. I wanted to be more attractive to all ladies when I started my journey. Now, all I care about is my personal happiness and appealing to her. Still, there are some things I'd like to mention about the comparison of me to others in regards to aging. I'm trying to summarize it without sounding vain but there really is no way to do that. I'm not as vain as I once was. My partner has commented on the improvement numerous times. Still, I need to mention how this effort has benefitted me with respect to others my age.

Before I met my friend, I attended a singles function with several people my age. The others had shown up earlier than me so I arrived after they had all been seated and visiting for a while. I noticed almost immediately that I was garnering attention from the ladies in the crowd over several of the males who had been there before me. Although the other males had engaged and I had yet to, there was a distinct level of attention focused on me by the ladies. Intrigued by this, I tried to get some information about the other males around me who looked older than I. As it turned out, they were within a few years of my age. We are not talking a few years older looking. Most of them looked to be in there seventies or more with gray hair, sagging, and wrinkles. I realized that this was due mostly to their appearance. Their bodies had sagged or were carrying extra weight compared to the more defined physique that I sported. Their skin was light and peaked looking compared to the tan that I had maintained through my outdoor activity. Their mannerisms were tired and slow whereas mine was upbeat and perky. They dressed more conservatively with baggy clothes whereas I sported tight clothes that hugged my body.

There was an apparent difference in the ages between myself and the other members. Each of the women at the function glanced at me more often and made an effort to talk to me while ignoring the others. I believe that my state of fitness was the reason for this. By being tanner and more fit, I looked younger. I also dressed for my body as did the others. The tighter clothes that I wore made a difference in the way I was perceived. It was apparent in the reactions and comments of the ladies.

My friend and owner of the weight loss facility where I had rented the room had informed me of this potential change. She said that women would notice the improvement and flock to me. I didn't believe it until it happened. When it did, I tried to understand the difference that set me apart. It was the fact that being fit and happy had made me feel younger and appear younger. I looked different and happier than the others which was more appealing to the single ladies. I dressed the part in a manner that made me look young and vibrant rather than old and conservative. I feel that keeping on this trajectory will keep me from aging as quickly. I also feel that it is worth mentioning as incentive for you to look younger. Being fit can set you apart from the crowd as it did for me. It can make you look younger, feel younger, dress younger, and age slower.

My final comment on aging has to do with sagging. Body parts sag with age. For me, I had developed man boobs or "moobs" as I call them. I was able to reverse this sagging by perking up my pectoral muscles with chest exercises. I also eliminated the overhang in my waist. By tightening this area I have a body that looks more like a young man than an old one. Men naturally sag in the abdominal area as they age. This can be offset or reduced with a lifestyle change.

Similarly, I have not developed the sagging skin on my body that many people develop with age. My face does reflect aging and wrinkles from the weight loss. Whether this lack of sagging body skin is due to my lifestyle change or genetic makeup I don't know. What I do know is that there is a marked difference between the way my body has aged compared to those near my age in years. Because I am encouraging you the reader to set yourself apart in appearance through a lifestyle change, I thought it might be useful to write about this difference in aging as it is very notable between me and those of a similar age. The active lifestyle has made me look younger. I hope you realize the same success from your lifestyle change.

My breathing and stamina have also improved. Now I take stairs two at a time without slowing down. Before, I'd get winded about half way up. Now I power to the top without stopping. I also seem to not be able to tire out my abdominals. Something else on my body usually bothers me first. I can't seem to tire my legs or my core abdominal muscles. It appears that after a certain point of fitness attainment. These muscles seem to want more versus complaining with pain as they did initially. Of course there are limits to everything in life. I just can't seem to find mine in my legs and abdominal muscles. My lungs seem to handle whatever I throw at them. I don't have to stop to catch my breath. I get to an elevated level of breathing that I can maintain for a half an hour. I do notice this is affected by a cold or after I've eaten certain foods that weigh me down. Otherwise, I'm a perpetual machine that age hasn't affected. Granted I'm not sprinting or operating at extremely high levels of activity. On the other hand I'm not having to adhere to the fragile recommendations that websites recommend for people my age. 50 plus is not as limiting as you might think it is as I have discovered. Age does not limit you as much as you might think. Aging can occur at a different rate that fitness seems to improve. These are the observations that have resulted from my effort.

10. THE JOURNEY CONTINUES

There is no real end to this book as there is no end to my lifestyle change. I am on a continuous journey without a destination. I have reached and surpassed many milestones. To set a destination would mean, that I am admitting there will eventually be a time where I have to give up my efforts to improve on being healthy and remaining fit. I hope that time never comes. I want to enjoy this journey until I take my last breath in a set of lungs that use their capacity to the fullest.

Although there is an end to this writing, I am planning future updates and improvements. I will be communicating these via my website at http://weight-loss-over-50.com. I am planning a fitness blog. I also plan to contribute to other websites and various social media venues such as youtube, Facebook, LinkedIn, and Twitter as well as whatever else arises as the latest internet fad. Please check back in when you can by visiting my website. I plan to continue my journey and invite you to continue with me.

I hope my tips help you to succeed with your weight loss journey and quest to improve your fitness!

APPENDIX

Weight lifting of dumb bells (with some machine work)

1. Chest and arms (Triceps)
   a. Presses at 6 different incline levels (45 lbs; 50 reps); front view

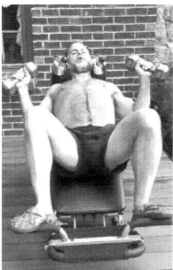

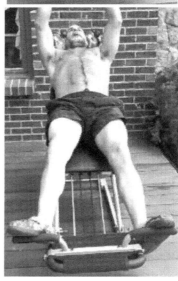

b. Presses at 6 different incline levels
    (45 lbs; 50 reps); side view

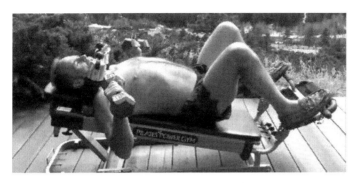

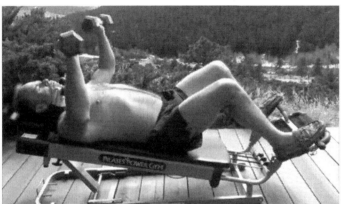

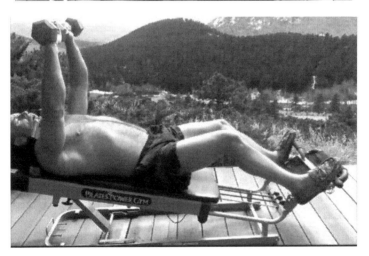

a. Presses at 3 different decline levels
    (45 lbs; 50 reps)

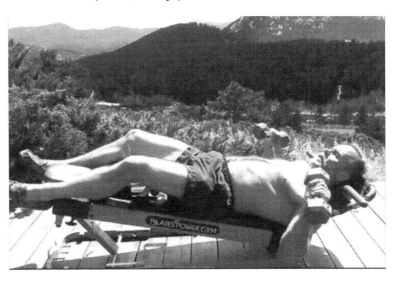

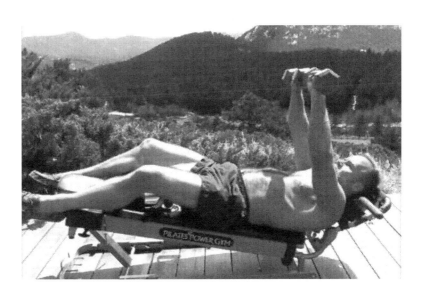

b. Flat presses (45 lbs; 50 reps)

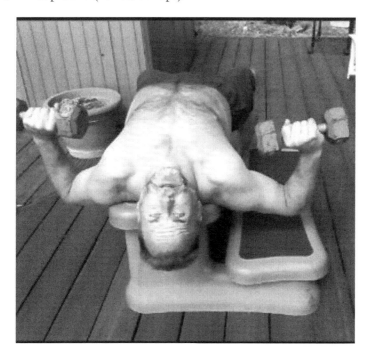

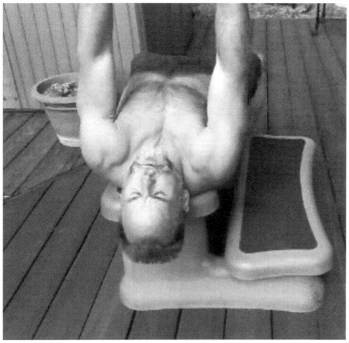

c. Above the head arm extensions
(20 lbs; 50 reps)

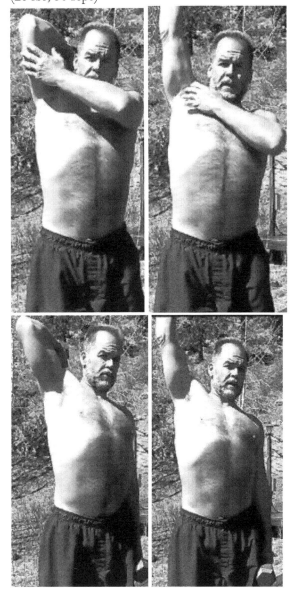

d. Level upper arm extensions
   (20 lbs; 50 reps)

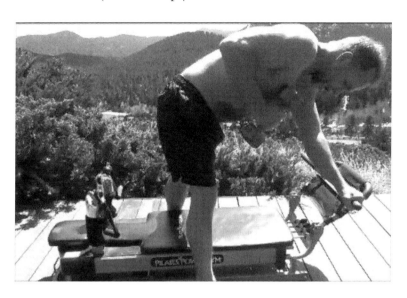

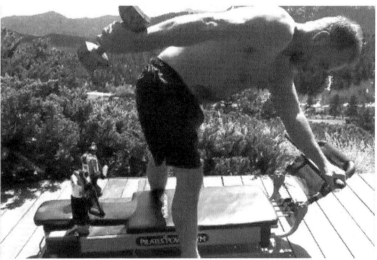

e. Extending the arms on the Pilates machine

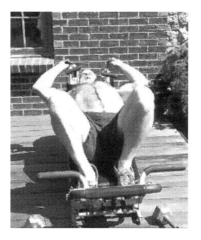

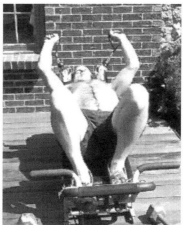

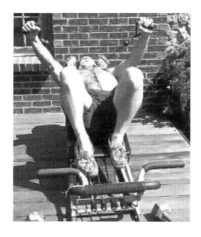

Extending the arms on the Pilates machine side view

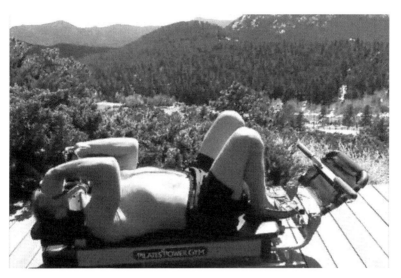

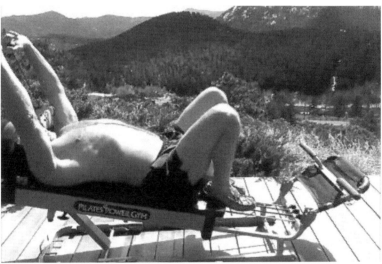

f.   Extending the arms on the flat bench with dumb bells

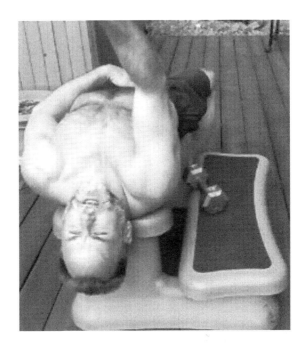

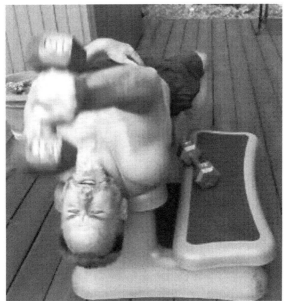

g.   Flies on a flat bench

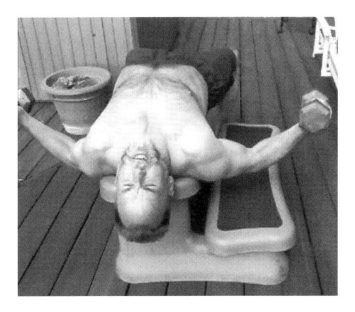

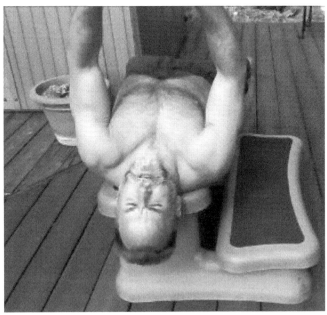

h. Pull overs

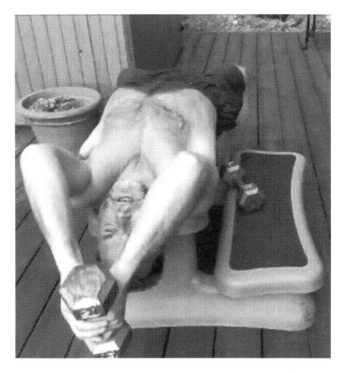

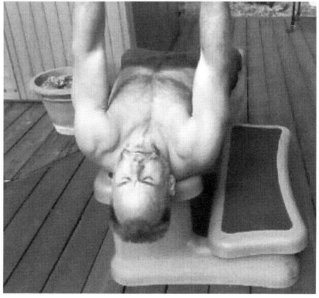

1. Shoulders (while wearing a weight belt for back support)
   a. Standing behind the back presses (45 lbs; 50 reps)

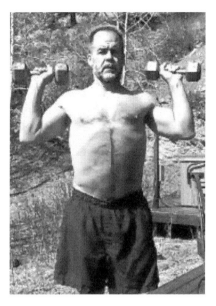

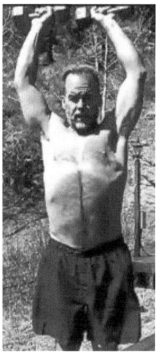

b.   Seated behind the back presses (45 lbs; 50 reps)

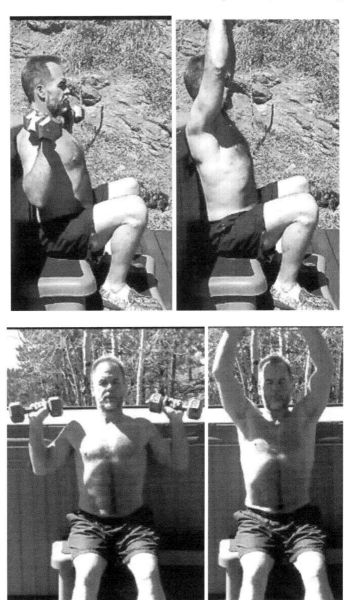

c.   Shrugs (45 lbs; 50 reps)

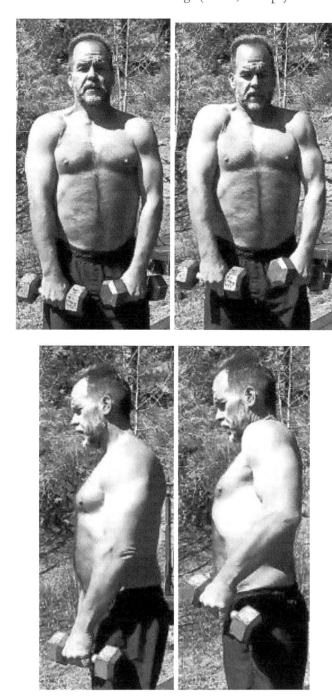

d. Upright rows (20 lbs; 50 reps)

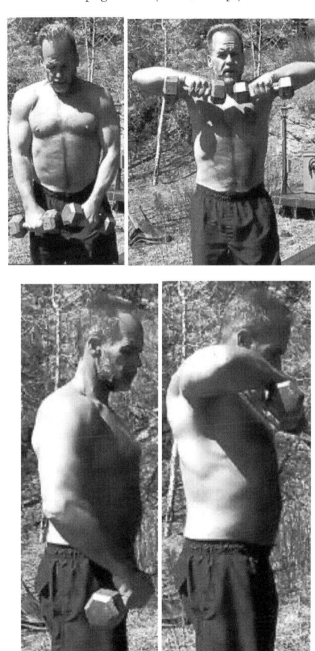

e.   Extended arm flies (side) (20 lbs; 50 reps

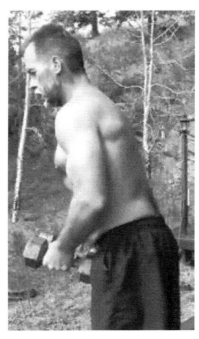

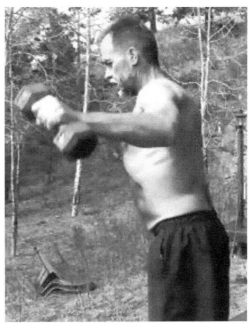

f.   Extended arm flies (front) (20 lbs; 50 reps)

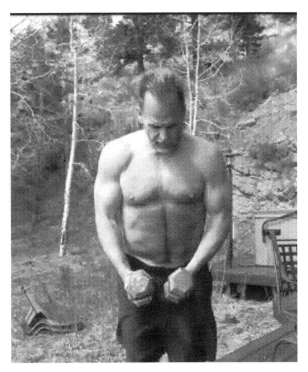

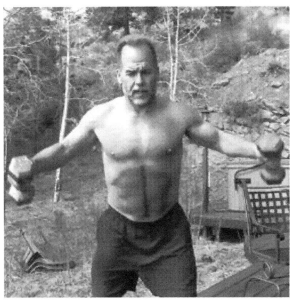

2. Back
    a. Rows on the Pilates machine (inclined)

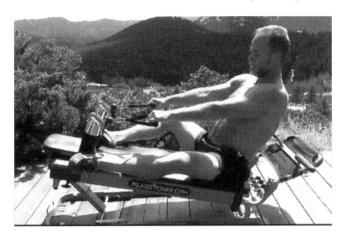

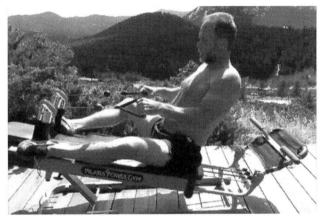

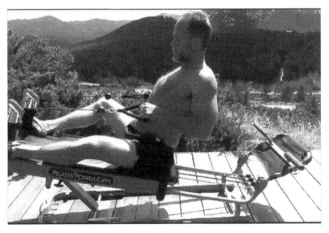

b.   Extended arm pull on the Pilates machine

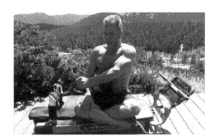

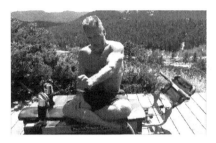

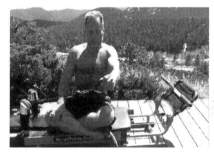

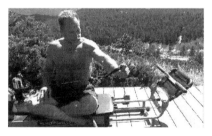

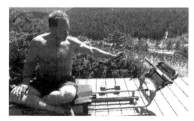

c.   Lat pull downs (side, inclined)

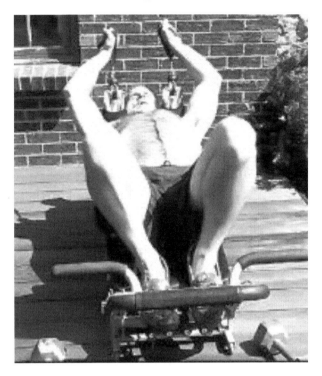

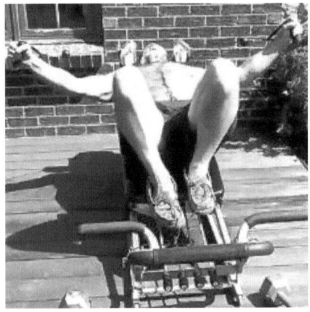

d.   Lat pull downs (front, inclined)

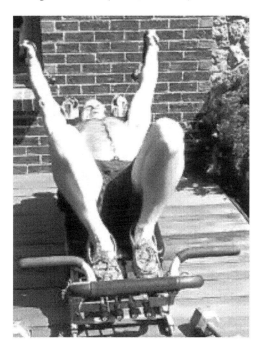

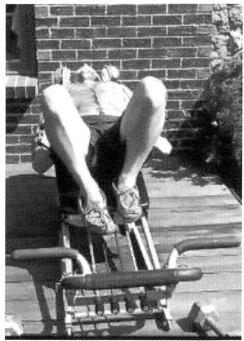

e. Bent over rows (45 lbs; 50 reps)

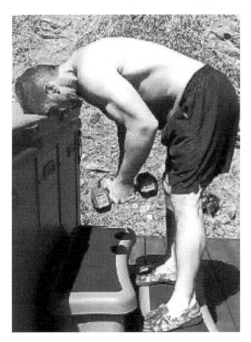

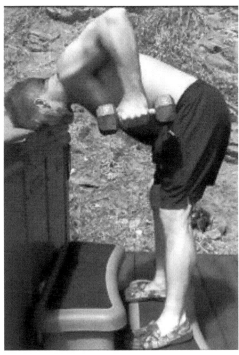

f.   Single arm pull (45 lbs; 50 reps)

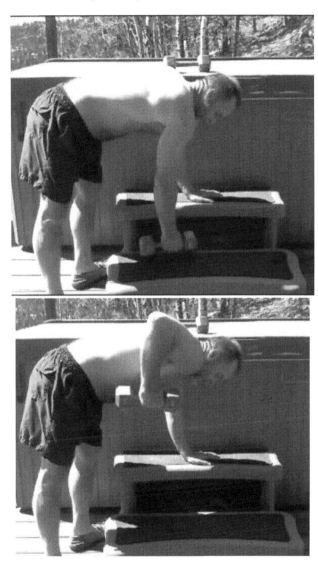

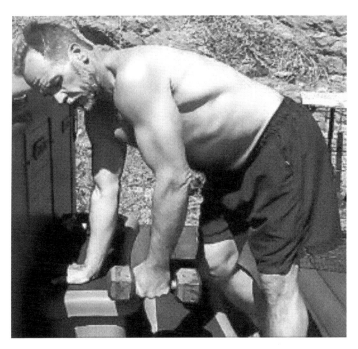

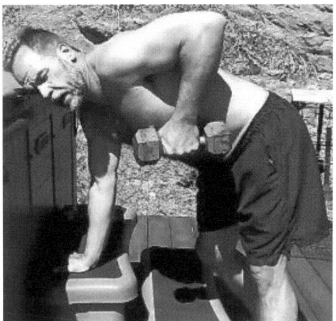

144

g. Standing back extension (45 lbs; 50 reps)

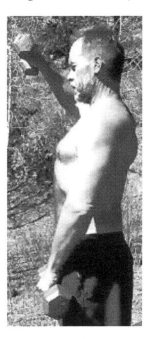

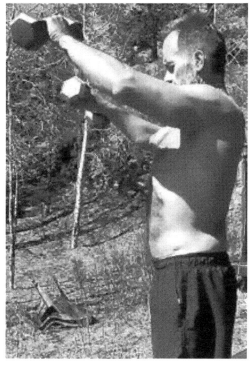

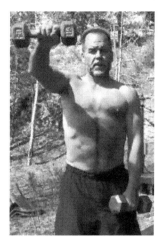

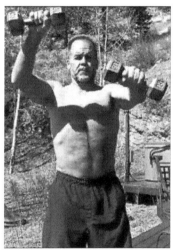

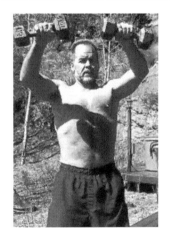

146

3. Biceps
   a.   Dumb bell curls

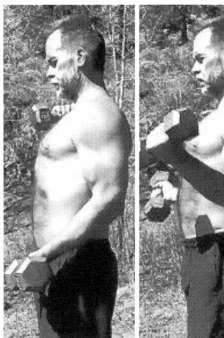

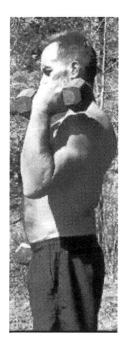

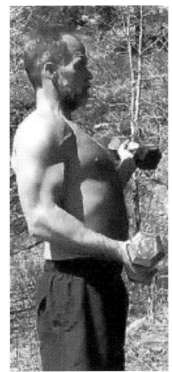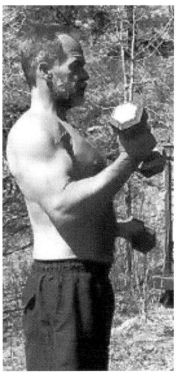

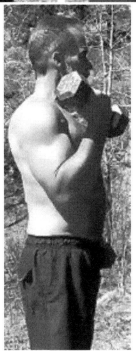

148

b. Pilates machine curls

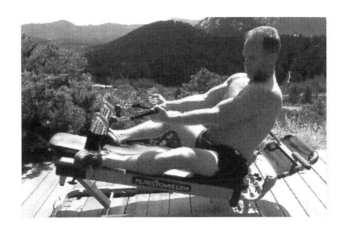

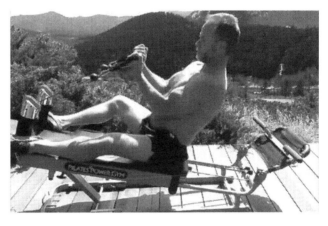

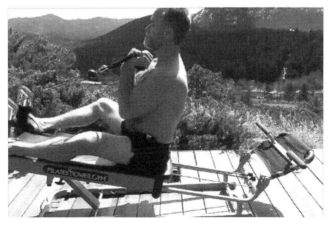

c. Stationary object curls

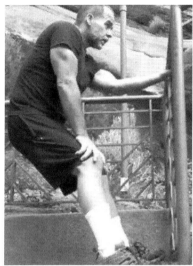
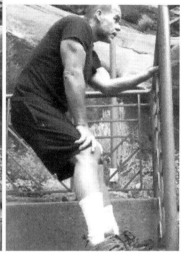
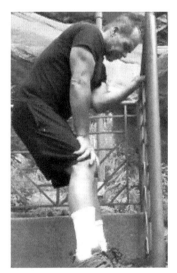

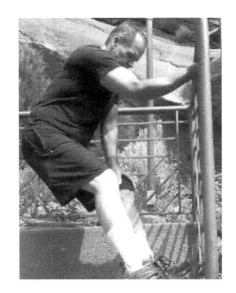

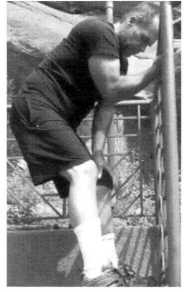
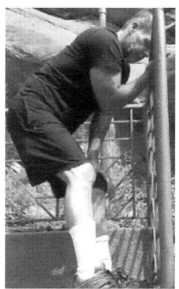

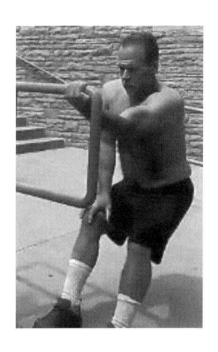

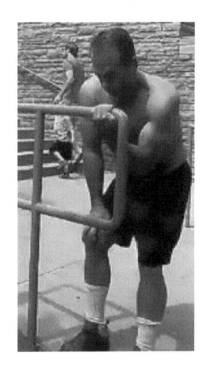

1. Full body dips

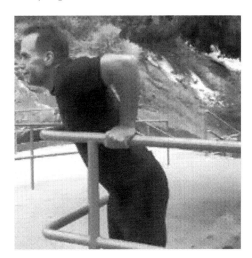

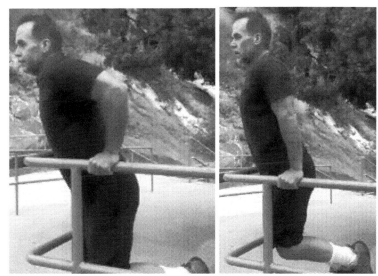

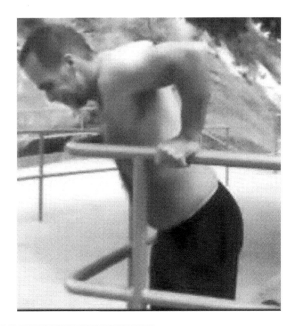

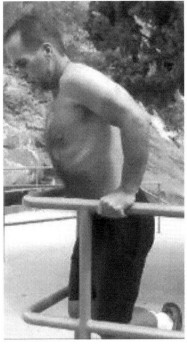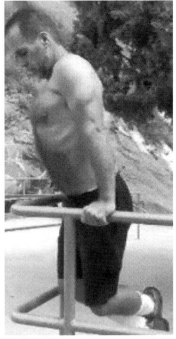

1. Half body dips

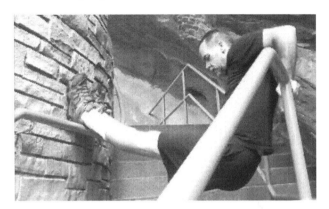

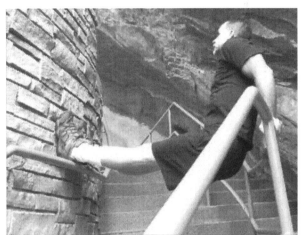

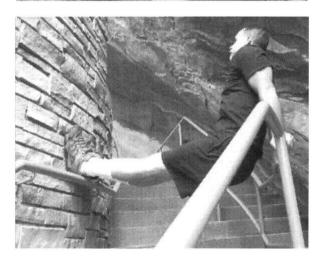

1. Leg lifts

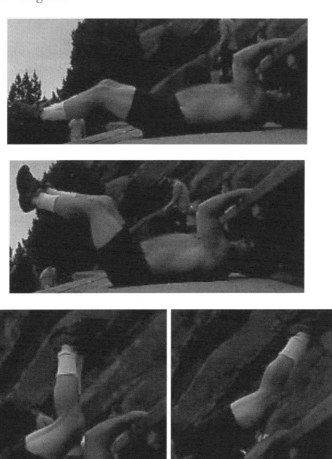

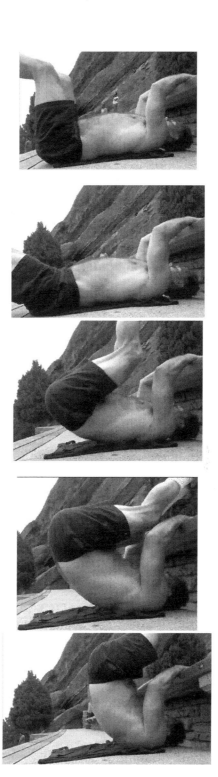

2. Pushups

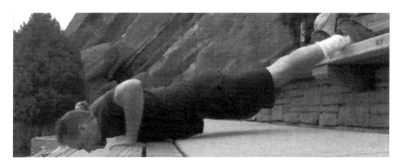

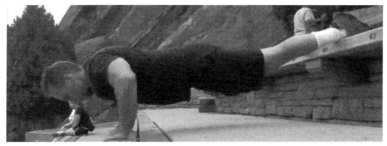

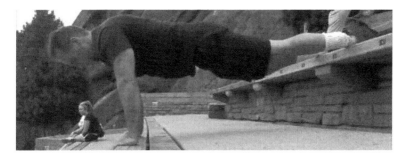

3. 100 side bends with a 45 pound dumb bell

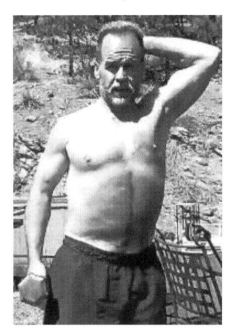

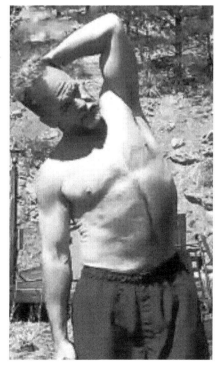

ABOUT THE AUTHOR

Scott Deuty is a normal guy that has tried to lose weight and keep it off on three separate occasions. On this his fourth attempt, he has succeeded in obtaining the best physique of his life at age 52.

Scott has been publishing his work for over twenty five years having written many technical articles and a trail guide. Scott has a publication on the internet that has lasted over 20 years on a technology that has grown dramatically. This Application Note (search AN1520) still has relevance today after being originally published in 1993. Scott was created the first known publication to overlay GPS coordinates on topographical maps in "The Four Wheel Drive Trails of Arizona". Scott's success is a testament to his ability as a visionary who sees developing trends in the marketplace and creates applicable written material. Scott also speaks publically and has training as a community college professor and off-road driving instructor.

In addition to this work, Scott has a fiction thriller novel in the works.

Scott holds a Master's Degree in Electrical Engineering from Virginia Tech, a Bachelor's Degree in Electrical Engineering from Syracuse University, and a Bachelor's Degree in Physics from the State University of New York at Geneseo.

Scott's websites include a variety of subject matter and are located at:

- http://phase-locked-loop.com,
- http://minimonstertruck.com,
- http://movealongs.com, and
- http://weight-loss-over-50.com.
- http://www.cafepress.com/stayhard

Made in the USA
Middletown, DE
02 August 2016